CRAFTS
IN
THERAPY AND
REHABILITATION

SECOND EDITION

CRAFTS
IN
THERAPY AND
REHABILITATION

SECOND EDITION

MARGARET DRAKE, PhD, OTR/L, ATR-BC, FAOTA

UNIVERSITY OF MISSISSIPPI MEDICAL CENTER

JACKSON, MISSISSIPPI

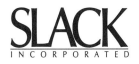

6900 GROVE ROAD, THOROFARE, NJ 08086-9447

Publisher: John H. Bond
Editorial Director: Amy E. Drummond
Associate Editor: Jennifer L. Stewart

Drake, Margaret
    Crafts in Therapy and Rehabilitation/Margaret Drake. -- 2nd ed.
        p. cm
    Includes bibliographical references and index.
    ISBN 1-55642-396-9 (alk. paper)
    1. Handicraft--Therapeutic use.   2. Occupational therapy.
I. Title.
    [DNLM: 1. Occupational Therapy--methods.   2. Art therapy--methods.
WB 555 D762c 1999}
RM735. 7.H35D73   1999
615.8'515--dc21
DNLM/DLC
for Library of Congress   98-42014

Printed in the United States of America

Published by: SLACK Incorporated
               6900 Grove Road
               Thorofare, NJ 08086-9447 USA
               Telephone: 609-848-1000
               Fax: 609-853-5991
               http://www.slackinc.com

Contact SLACK Incorporated for more information about other books in this field or about the availability of our books from distributors outside the United States.

Last digit is print number: 10 9 8 7 6 5 4 3 2 1

DEDICATION

This second edition is dedicated to the faculty and students
who used the first edition and shared with the author
what was important and what needed to be added.

CONTENTS

ACKNOWLEDGMENTS

I want to acknowledge the following people for their input and assistance in revising *Crafts in Therapy and Rehabilitation*: Kim Curbow-Wilcox, MS, PT, my officemate who willingly shared her knowledge of neuromotor behavioral theories and issues. Sandy Lowman, the Occupational Therapy Department head secretary who assisted me with a variety of technical challenges. For the first edition, I wrote the book by hand and gave it to a secretary to be typed. This time, I typed the text and revisions myself. Sandy helped me navigate the morass of new technology needed to do this. Joyce Titus, MPH, OTR/L, who liberally shared her experiences of using the first edition of *Crafts* and her ideas about how to better meet the needs of students and beginning therapists. Cyndi Scott, MBA, PT, who shared her knowledge of stroke, as did Marcia King, MEd, OTR/L, Peter Fayard, MA, OTR/L, and Amanda Bowen, OTR/L. Dr. Kathy Steen and Mr. Bob Howle provided excellent help in updating the chapter on computer crafts. For the new chapter on home health and found materials, Carol Tubbs, MA, OTR/L, shared her knowledge of home health from her years of experience in delivering care in that setting. She also used her excellent English skills to proof-read parts of this revision. Peter Giroux, MA, OTR/L, freely shared his books on pediatrics and development. Amy Drummond and Debra Christy at SLACK Incorporated have worked with me in a way that has been affirming. Lastly, I want to thank my department chair, Bette Groat, MA, OTR/L, and Dean Maury Mahan, PhD, for providing a supportive setting in which to do this work. There are any number of other individuals who have helped in other ways too, such as my students, who have encouraged me through this process. Books such as this do not happen through the efforts of just one person, but through the support and open sharing of knowledge and experience of many people. I want to thank all those who were involved.

—*Margaret Drake, PhD, OTR/L, ATR-BC, FAOTA*

PREFACE

With the world of knowledge expanding and multiplying at such a rapid rate, it is not really possible to keep perfectly current. However, as the profession of occupational therapy is adapting to the changing worldwide health care delivery system, new ways of looking at ideas and new ways of using language evolve. It may seem that it is impossible to keep up with the flow of new information, but it is important to remember that knowledge is not final. We continually add to what we know and adapt old knowledge to new learning. Each publication is part of the history we are writing about our profession. Therefore, this second edition is just one spot on the path of learning how to use crafts with patients. Hopefully it incorporates the knowledge that has developed since its first edition. Let us continue to enjoy crafts with our patients.

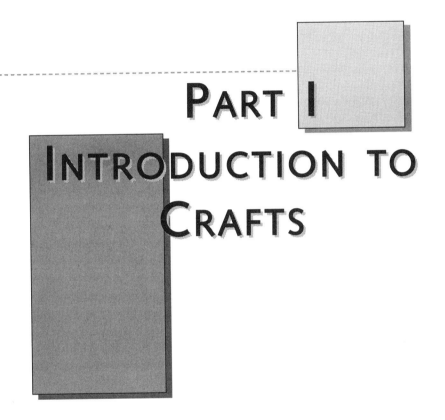

PART I
INTRODUCTION TO CRAFTS

THERAPEUTIC USE OF CRAFTS: WHAT ARE CRAFTS?

Craft (kraft): an occupation requiring special skill;
especially any of the manual arts
(*Webster's New World Dictionary*, 1982).

Why is the use of crafts in occupational therapy a topic to be explored? In this time of shortened hospital stays and limited resources for supply and equipment budgets, therapists are forced to streamline their treatment procedures. Information technology products such as computers and videos, which have thrust us into the current information age, have also carried us away from and obscured the usefulness of one of our very useful modalities of occupational therapy treatment: crafts. We have moved toward more frequent use of electronic media in client treatment, such as computers and videos, and while that may not diminish the emphasis on what we do with our hands and bodies, the reality is there is so little time available for treatment of clients that therapists must choose among treatment modalities, and many choose computers.

Additionally, in a work-oriented culture like ours, crafts have come to symbolize a leisure time activity rather than real work. As medical diagnostic and treatment technology has mushroomed, occupational therapy has been forced to appear more scientific. Somehow, crafts seem not so scientific. Even as early as 1924, the Boston School of Occupational Therapy defined our profession with emphasis on the scientific and measurable use of activities to achieve reduction of dysfunction (Reed, 1983). However, as in medicine, in which physicians are realizing that quality time spent interviewing/listening to a client produces as much information as more expensive tests and procedures, occupational therapists are realizing that our traditional methods also produce valuable results.

While use of crafts in therapy has changed (Taylor, Manguna, 1991), more than half of all occupational therapy clinics treating pediatric, geriatric, physically dysfunctional, and mentally ill clients continue to use basic crafts such as leatherwork and needlework in treatment. A recent survey of fieldwork sites verifies this (Titus, 1997). Certainly, as many therapists use crafts and make splints.

As our literature has developed over the last 25 years, the word *crafts* has been almost obliterated from the professional vocabulary. The two most recent comprehensive occupational therapy texts (Neistadt, Crepeau, 1997; Christiansen, Baum, 1997) have no listing for crafts in their indices. Rather than saying "craft session," we say *task group* (Fidler, 1984) or *dyadic interaction skills group* (Arbesman, et al, 1984). Task group is a term that came into use in the later 1960s (Fidler, 1969). Early photographs in *A Functional Approach to Group Work in Occupational Therapy*, by Howe and Schwartzberg (Howe, Schwartzberg, 1986), have titles of task groups and project groups when what they were doing were crafts. Textbooks from the last 60 years show how the terminology related to crafts has changed. This is described in more detail later in this chapter. We need to continue to revalue for ourselves the usefulness of craft media in treatment (Fidler, Fidler, 1981).

Crafts in particular help clients realize that through the process of taking raw materials or minimally prepared substances and processing, assembling, and forming them, the clients can do the same with their lives. Crafts are a microcosm of life—one receives basic raw materials and through a series of efforts, waiting periods, and guidance, one lives a life—one creates a craft product. Crafts are a teaching example of how to put it all together. This concept makes crafts valuable therapeutic media for the modern clinical setting with short hospital stays.

As we learn more about brain lateralization and localized specialization, we know that crafts are able to naturally use the spatial and intuitive functions of the nondominant side of the brain (Miller, 1988a; Miller, 1988b; Ornstein, 1988; Rosenfeld, 1988; Leask, Crow, 1997). As a profession, we have intuitively understood that crafts help use and rehabilitate brain functions, but we did not know why.

Now this information is gradually being authenticated through research (Corballis, Beals, 1983; Herrmann, 1988; Boucher, Bryden, 1997; Thibodaux, Ludwig, 1988). There is scientific evidence to show why crafts perform rehabilitative functions more efficiently than exercise or other occupations (Lin, 1997; Stancliff, 1996). While use of crafts cannot do everything, they are important and valid treatment media. We do not want to go back to a time when there were only a few treatment modalities—crafts being the main one. It is important to keep crafts as one of many treatment alternatives.

A look at the indices and tables of contents of the profession's textbooks over the years gives a little insight into how crafts were viewed. The very first edition of *Occupational Therapy,* by Willard and Spackman (1947), lists seven crafts under activities in the index. The word *handicrafts* was used to define another 18 items. All but one of the 15 photographs show a craft in progress. The second edition, *Principles of Occupational Therapy* (1954), does not use the word crafts in the index, but under activities, lists 14 separate crafts. The title of a section of the chapter *Activities in Occupational Therapy* is "Handicrafts."

Most of the "Activities Suggested to Provide Treatment" in the third edition (Willard, Spackman, 1963) are crafts; however, a glance through the table of contents and index gives almost no hint that crafts are a major activity or occupation. By the fourth edition (1971), under activities in the index, no crafts are named, but when one turns to the page for "Activities for Restoration of Function," most of the activities/occupations listed are indeed crafts. In the fifth edition (Hopkins, Smith, 1978), one must search to find any allusion to crafts. Euphemisms such as *functional activities* or *avocational activities* are used instead. The sixth edition (1983) contains one paragraph entitled "To Use Crafts or Not to Use Crafts?" This 1983 text lists leather lacing, woodworking, and crafts with *therapeutic use* in the index. The seventh edition (1988) reflects the increased use of computer technology with 11 index listings for computers and one for crafts as therapy. Throughout the chapter on historical perspectives, attitudes toward crafts by the profession's leaders are mentioned. In the eighth edition (1993), crafts are only named in components of assessments, and photographs show formal assessments that have taken pieces of crafts and isolated them as an evaluation tool. The ninth edition (Neistadt, Crepeau, 1997) has photographs of *expressive activities* such as art, dance, and expressive crafts.

Another text, *Prescribing Occupational Therapy,* by Dr. William Dunton (1945), emphasizes the prescription from physicians for occupational therapy treatment. This book tells how the therapist may be in a better position than the physician to choose activities. A 10-page section gives "Suggestions of the Use of Crafts in Functional Restoration," plus a 15-item guide for selection that emphasizes craft quality and usefulness.

Finally, in 1991, a comprehensive occupational therapy textbook competing with the Willard and Spackman series was published, *Occupational Therapy: Overcoming Performance Deficits* (Christiansen, Baum, 1991). Case studies describe clients involved in crafts by euphemisms such as *hobbies* and *the arts,* which are used rather than the more concrete word—crafts. The second edition of this new text appeared in 1997. Crafts are mentioned incidental to their use as assessments (i.e., Draw-A-Person test, Allen Cognitive Levels Assessment, and Lerner's Magazine Picture Collage).

Many books currently being used that one would assume would mention crafts do not list them in the index (Bruce, Borg, 1993; Christiansen, 1994; Lohman, Padilla, Byers-Connon, 1998). On the other hand, other texts reflect the value of crafts and do list them (Cynkin, Robinson, 1990;

Early, 1993; Cottrell, 1996). This exemplified the ambivalence felt by many occupational therapists to these modalities, which are used in many clinics. Barris, Kielhofner, and Watts (1988) attribute the diminishing discussion of crafts in occupational therapy "to the general devaluation of handmade objects in American culture." In a 1986 (Barris, Kielhofner, Watts, 1988) and 1988 study, which Barris collaborated on, and a 1997 study by Titus (Barris, Cordero, Christiaansen, 1986), cooking was found to be the most commonly used craft. Therapists answering the surveys worked in physical disabilities, mental health, pediatrics, developmental disabilities, hand clinics, geriatrics, and institutions that treat the whole range of disabilities. A 1989 unpublished survey from Florida International University on "what crafts are being taught in occupational therapy programs" found a similar ranking of which crafts are used more often: woodworking, leather, needlework, copper tooling, mosaics, and ceramics, followed by a number of other crafts. The chapters of this book are organized around this frequency ranking with the more frequently used crafts coming first.

Associations of pottery and weaving with goddess worship have been suggested as evidence that these crafts were invented by women (Eisler, 1987). Many crafts were invented by women to assist them in their primary role as mother and nurturer. Early woodworking and leathercraft for women would have included making cradles and cradleboards to carry babies on their backs while they went to gather food or tend to animals. We know that in hunter-gatherer cultures, men killed and brought home game, and women prepared the hides (Boserup, 1970; Morgan, 1972; Rich, 1976; Danday, 1981) and sewed them together for clothes, shelter, and food containers. With the development of metal, men began to take over some crafts as they developed more efficient weapons and warfare. As patriarchy prevailed, men took over many prestigious crafts such as woodworking and pottery. When the industrial revolution swept away many handicrafts, those that remained, like needlework and china painting, again became the province of women (Boserup, 1970; Morgan, 1972; Rich, 1976; Danday, 1981; Whyte, 1978; Sochen, 1974). While men continued to dominate woodworking, leathercraft, and pottery in western culture, possibly the decline in status for some crafts has to do with their identification with women.

Historically, documentation of crafts in health treatment is sketchy until the latter 18th century; however, music as treatment is commonly mentioned among the ancients (Willard, Spackman, 1947). In earlier times, as noted above, crafts were undoubtedly a necessity for clothing, food containers, implements, and tools. Something so integral to daily life may not have had the healing properties that we attribute to crafts today. However, Rich (1976) credits early arts such as weaving and pottery with magical qualities, although rituals and taboos among primitive peoples have been given more credit than crafts for cures (Achternecht, 1971).

Galen, the Greek physician who adopted Rome as his home, did recommend exercise (MacKenzie, 1979) and felt that clients are healed by being occupied (Willard, Spackman, 1954); however, he did not specify crafts. The Arabs adopted much of what was good from Greek and Roman medicine. Ibn Jazlah, an Arabic physician in the Middle Ages (500 to 1500 AD), recommended physical treatments such as baths and exercise (Granziani, 1980). Some tribes of Native Americans, such as the Navaho and Cheyenne, have traditionally used painting and sand painting in healing and medicine (Achternecht, 1971).

In Europe during the Middle Ages, enlightened and humane client treatment for most disorders was eclipsed. With the development of humane treatment of clients in Europe at the beginning of the 19th century, Phillipe Pinel persuaded tradesmen in Paris to give craftwork to his clients in Aisle de Bicetre. Throughout Europe, similar developments in humane treatment followed (Pinel, 1806).

About the same time, Dr. Benjamin Rush, a signer of the Declaration of Independence and father of American psychiatry, used work and some crafts with this clients at Pennsylvania Hospital in Philadelphia (Willard, Spackman, 1954; Haworth, MacDonald, 1946). By mid-century, clients' craftwork was being advertised for sale in London (Haworth, MacDonald 1946). Up through the latter part of the 19th century, many mental hospitals developed programs that included occupations, amusements, and crafts.

Probably the first professional writing occupational therapists have on crafts in treatment is *Studies in Invalid Occupations* (Tracy, 1910). The author, Susan Tracy, was the first to designate specific crafts for specific needs. From then on, publications in occupational therapy included instructions on how to use crafts to treat clients. The refinement of skills in choosing the best occupation or activity for each client continues. This book further presents the use of crafts in health care for an era in which faster is better and competition and quantity production are the emphasized, valued ethic and norm rather than quality, hand-crafted articles.

REFERENCES

Achternecht, E. H. (1971). *Medicine and ethnology: Elements and exercises.* Lawrence, KS: The University of Kansas Press.

Arbesman, F., et al. (1984). *Occupational therapy: Protocols in mental health.* Baltimore: Betty Cox Associates.

Barris, R., Cordero, J., & Christiaansen, R. (1986). Occupational therapist's use of media *Am J Occup Ther, 40*(10), 679-684.

Barris, R., Kielhofner, G., & Watts, J. (1988). *Occupational therapy in psychosocial practice.* Thorofare, NJ: SLACK Incorporated.

Boserup, E. (1970). *Women's role in economic development.* London: George Allen and Unwin.

Boucher, R., & Bryden, M. P. (1997). Lateality effects in the processing of melody and timbre. *Neuropsychologia, 35*(11), 1467-1473.

Bruce, M. A., & Borg, B. (1993). *Psychosoocial occupational therapy: Frames of reference for intervention* (2nd ed.). Thorofare, NJ: SLACK Incorporated.

Christiansen, C. ed. (1994). *Ways of living: Self-care strategies for special needs,* Rockville, MD: American Occupational Therapy Association.

Christiansen, C., & Baum, C. (1991). *Occupational therapy: Overcoming human performance deficits.* Thorofare, NJ: SLACK Incorporated.

Christiansen, C., & Baum, C. (1997). *Occupational therapy: Enabling function and well-being* (2nd ed.). Thorofare, N.J.: SLACK Incorporated.

Corballis, M., & Beals, I. (1983). *The ambivalent mind.* Chicago: Nelson-Hall.

Cottrell, R. P. F. (1996). *Perspectives on purposeful activity: Foundation & future of occupational therapy.* Bethesda, MD: American Occupational Therapy Association.

Cynkin, S., & Robinson, A. M. (1990). *Occupational health and activities health: Toward health through activities.* Boston: Little, Brown, and Co.

Danday, P. R. (1981). *Female power and male dominance: On the origin of sexual inequality.* Cambridge: Cambridge University Press.

Dunton, W. R. (1945). *Prescribing occupational therapy* (2nd ed.). Springfield, IL: Charles C. Thomas.

Early, M. B. (1993). *Mental health concepts and techniques for the occupational therapy assistant* (2nd ed.). New York: Raven Press.

Eisler, R. (1987). *The chalice and the blade.* New York: Harper and Row.

Fidler, G. S. (1969). The task-oriented group as a context for treatment. *Am J Occup Ther, 23*(1), 43-48.

Fidler, G. S. (1984). *Designs of rehabilitation services in psychiatric hospital settings.* Laurel, MD: Ramsco Publishing Co.

Fidler, G. S., & Fidler, J. W. A. (1981). From crafts to competence. *Am J Occup Ther, 35*(9), 567-573.

Florida International University. (1989). Unpublished material.

Granziani, J. S. (1980). *Arabic medicine in the eleventh century as represented in the works of Ibn Jazlah.* Karachi, Pakistan: Hamard Academy Press.

Haworth, N. A., & MacDonald, E. M. (1946). *Theory of occupational therapy.* Baltimore: Williams and Wilkins.

Herrmann, N. (1988). *The creative brain.* Lake Lure, NC: Applied Creative Services.

Hopkins, H. L., & Smith, H. D. (1978). *Willard and Spackman's occupational therapy* (5th ed.). Philadelphia: Lippincott.

Hopkins, H. L., & Smith, H. D. (1983). *Willard and Spackman's occupational therapy* (6th ed.). Philadelphia: Lippincott.

Hopkins, H. L., & Smith, H. D. (1988). *Willard and Spackman's occupational therapy* (7th ed.). Philiadelphia: Lippincott.

Hopkins, H. L., & Smith, H. D. (1993). *Willard and Spackman's occupational therapy* (8th ed.). Philadelphia: Lippincott.

Howe, M., & Schwartzberg, S. (1986). *A functional approach to group work in occupational therapy.* Philadelphia: Lippincott.

Leask, S. J., & Crow, T. J. (1997). How far does the brain lateralize?: an unbiased method for determining the optimum degree of hemispheric specialization. *Neuropsychologia, 35*(10), 1381-1387.

Lin, K. C. (1997). Enhancing occupational performance through occupationally embedded exercise: A meta-analytic review. *The Occupational Therapy Journal of Research, 17*(11), 25-47

Lohman, H., Padilla, R. L., & Byers-Connon, S. (1998). *Occupational therapy with elders.* St. Louis: Mosby.

MacKenzie, J. (1979). *The history of health and art of preserving it.* New York: Arno Press.

Miller, L. (1988a). The emotional brain. *Psychology Today, 22*(2), 34-42.

Miller, L. (1988b). Men without passion. *Psychology Today, 22*(12), 20-22.

Morgan, E. (1972). *The Descent of Women.* New York: Stein and Day.

Neistadt, M. E., & Crepeau E. B. (1997). *Willard and Spackman's occupational therapy* (9th ed.). Philadelphia: Lippincott.

Ornstein, R. E. (1972). *The Psychology of Consciousness.* San Francisco: W. H. Freeman and Company.

Pinel, P. (1806). *Traite medico-philosophique de l'alienation mentale.* Paris: J. A. Brosson.

Reed, K. L., & Sanderson, S. R. (1983). *Concepts of occupational therapy* (2nd ed.). Baltimore: Williams & Wilkins.

Rich, A. (1976). *Of Women Born.* New York: Bantam Books.

Rosenfeld, A. A. (1988). New images, new insights into your brain. *Psychology Today, 22*(11), 22-24.

Sochen, J. (1974). *Herstory: A woman's view of American history.* New York: Alfred Publishing Co.

Stancliff, B. L. (1996). Roundtable: Are arts and crafts a valuable modality? *OT Practice, 1*(10), 51-54.

Taylor, E., & Manguna, J. (1991). Use of treatment activities in occupational therapy. *Am J Occup Ther, 45*(4), 317-322.

Thibodaux, C. S., & Ludwig, F. M. (1988). Intrinsic movement in product oriented and non-product oriented activities. *Am J Occup Ther, 42*(3), 169-175

Titus, J. (1997) Treatment interventions used on level II occupational therapy fieldwork. Unpublished manuscript.

Tracy, S. (1910). *A manual for nurses and attendants: Studies in invalid occupations.* Boston: Whitcomb Barrows.

Webster's New World Dictionary, 2nd College Edition. (1982).

Whyte, M. K. (1978). *The status of women in preindustrial societies.* Princeton, NJ: Princeton University Press.

Willard, H. S., & Spackman, C. S. (1947). *Principles of occupational therapy.* Philadelphia: Lippincott.

Willard, H. S., & Spackman, C. S. (1954). *Principles of occupational therapy* (2nd ed.). Philadelphia: Lippincott.

Willard, H. S., & Spackman, C. S. (1963). *Occupational therapy* (3rd ed.). Philadelphia: Lippincott.

Willard, H. S., & Spackman, C. S. (1971). *Occupational therapy* (4th ed.). Philadelphia: Lippincott.

THEORIES TO RATIONALIZE CHOICE OF PURPOSEFUL ACTIVITY

INTRODUCTION

Much has been written and discussed over the past two decades regarding naming and categorizing theories by which occupational therapists operate. Dr. Gary Kielhofner, one of our foremost theoreticians proposes, "that the paradigm is the cultural core of the discipline" of occupational therapy (1997). The paradigm of occupational therapy states that activities and occupations assist in healing. Clients who are self-motivated or can be motivated by an occupational therapist to participate in activities and occupations will enhance their chances of improving their function and state of well-being.

The next level of theory is the practice models. These correspond to what some think of as the frames of reference (Kielhofner, 1997). Kielhofner, along with the writers of the 1991 American Occupational Therapy Association Accreditation Committee Essentials, use the term "models" to differentiate "the theories of human adaptation," which therapists use to explain the reason they choose certain modalities (AOTA, 1991). Each model is based on a theory. A theory is an idea about why life is like it is and why things and people work the way they work. "Theory is not static, nor is it ever final" (Llorens, 1984). Humans are continuously refining and changing their thinking. Occupational therapy theory is thus changing continuously as therapists create new ideas about the humans they work with and how they respond to therapy. Often different occupational therapy theories have elements in common that make it hard for clinicians to differentiate one from another.

When authors choose different models to include in their books and articles, each chooses those which appear to have the most important and relevant ideas at the time of writing. In this information age in which new ideas are quickly discussed, analyzed, and published, it is difficult to know which theories will continue to be used and which will emerge and disappear. Sometimes different names are given to models that appear to be essentially the same. In the interest of simplicity and clarity, only the models from *Willard and Spackman's Occupational Therapy*, ninth edition (1997), Kielhofner's *Conceptual Foundations of Occupational Therapy*, second edition (1997), Christiansen and Baum's *Occupational Therapy: Enabling Function and Well-Being*, second edition (1997), and Fidler in the *American Journal of Occupational Therapy* (1996), have been included in this text. Not all models mentioned in these texts and periodicals are named here. Theories with a similar theoretical base and view of humanity, illness, and occupation are grouped under one heading. The ideas of some occupational therapists may have contributed to more than one model. In this book, the term *occupation* is synonymous with *crafts*. Whenever possible, other previous "frames of reference" that relate to the model described here will be included so that the student can identify which theories belong together. The central objective of this chapter is to simplify occupational therapy theories to make it easier to apply them to crafts.

Models are based on concepts and principles about how to work with particular problems. For example, a person who operated on the principle that all development of morals takes place before age 6 will have a different approach to teen and adult clients than a person who believes in the concept that humans are always learning and growing morally. The first person might strongly believe in incarceration and punishment while the second would believe in providing many learning and growing experiences. The first person might use certain crafts as punishment or might deprive the client of crafts as punishment. The second person may want to use only crafts that would provide new learning for clients or that could provide altruistic experiences such as making toys for a children's hospital. The principles underlying each approach would greatly affect which crafts were offered, which tools were allowed, the context or where they might be used, and almost every other aspect of the decision-making process. Therefore, the models that give meaning to these concepts and principles become very important to the individual therapist. For this reason, the student needs to evaluate and compare the concepts and principles underlying each model.

NEUROMOTOR BEHAVIOR MODEL

Human function is made up of a balance of biochemical and biological processes. The function of each human is expressed in the integration of sensory input and perceptual-motor output. This input-output process constitutes demonstrated behavior. Movement and the behavior that results from movement of body parts is based on neurological wiring, chemical transport, and storage of information in the neurological system. Illness or defects in the brain, vestibular, proprioceptive visual, and auditory systems that interfere with awareness or in processing and integration of sensations in these systems may cause abnormal behavior. If a person has unusual movement patterns, it is considered to be the consequence of neurological transmission problems, muscular imbalance, or orthopedic structural distortion. This model is a combination of several well-known theories: neurodevelopmental treatment (Eggers, 1984), sensory integration (Fisher, Murray, Bundy, 1991; Van Deusen, 1993), myofacial release (Umphred, 1995), Brunnstrom (Trombly, 1995), motor control and learning (Neistadt, Crepeau, 1997; Montgomery, Connolly, 1991; Cohen, 1993; Carr, Shepherd, Gordon, Gentile, Held, 1987), proprioceptive neuromuscular facilitation (Umphred, 1995; Trombly, 1995; Cohen, 1993), and pharmacology (Bonder, 1991).

Occupational therapy treatment attempts to reverse the illness or defect. Making an impact on the neurological system often becomes the goal of treatment. It may be achieved by occupations that involve gross motor body movements. Heavy work patterns are considered normalizers of neurotransmitter balance in the neural system. Such activities also metabolize stress hormones and reduce abnormal feelings and reactions (Ayers, 1987). Crafts that involve heavy work patterns and postural changes are often considered most likely to achieve normal neural reactions. Sawing, hammering, throwing, and mixing can be used to achieve goals in this model.

LEARNING/COGNITIVE DISABILITIES

Humans are defined by their cognitive abilities, which are demonstrated in their ability to learn, speak, use language, and change and preserve material objects. Symbols, words, and language are important in assessing cognition and level of arousal. According to this model, illness or dysfunction means inability to learn or remember how to speak and how to do things. This model assumes that there is a relationship between biological abnormalities and psychiatric disease. Mental illness is considered to include impairment in sensory information processing (Kielhofner, 1997; Allen, 1985; Bruce, 1994; Katz, 1992). Learning in this model includes learning new behaviors.

One important function of the occupational therapist in the learning/cognitive disabilities model is to assess a client's cognitive function by observing task performance. In planning treatment, challenging activities beyond the client's current functioning are avoided. The client's ability to work with materials may change. The therapist must be attentive to these changes and provide the appropriate activities.

A variety of craft materials and activities is considered appropriate for different cognitive problems (Radomski, Dougherty, Fine, Baum, 1994; Earhart, Allen, 1988). Some publications on cognitive disabilities name specific crafts that are appropriate for different cognitive problems (Earhart, Allen, 1988, Earhart, Allen, Blue, 1993). The Allen Cognitive Levels (ACL) test involved leather lacing (Allen, Earhart, Blue, 1992).

DEVELOPMENTAL/SPATIOTEMPORAL ADAPTATION

In the developmental/spatiotemporal adaptation model, humans are assumed to progress in an orderly way through various growth stages. The changes may be gradual and a person may show behaviors from several different stages at the same time. Different theorists have described these stages with varying emphasis and time parameters (Case-Smith, Allen, Pratt, 1996; Gilfoyle, Grady, Moore, 1990; Kramer, Hinojosa, 1993). Illness or dysfunction is shown by the absence of age-appropriate behaviors. In other words, the sick client fails to pass through the expected stages of development or regresses from a higher to a lower stage. Dysfunction may be caused by neurological impairment, trauma, or environmental deficits. The cause is not as important as the effect on developmental function. Dysfunction is defined as the failure to master or accomplish the life tasks expected of that particular stage of development.

Occupations such as crafts are thought of primarily as vehicles for attaining stage-specific behavior, for achieving mastery of a developmental stage. The treatment environment is arranged to maximize and promote development. For example, for a dysfunctional 5-year-old, appropriate life tasks might include learning to get along in groups, copying letters, coloring within lines, using scissors, and constructing materials.

An appropriate developmental environment would include materials such as wood, hammer and nails, clay, paper for copying words from many large-print posters on the wall, and outline drawings of familiar objects to be colored, cut out, and pasted. Such activities would be carried out in dyads or small groups to accomplish the task of age-appropriate socialization (Neistadt, Crepeau, 1997; Duncome, Howe, Schwartzberg, 1988; Reed, 1984; Reed, Sanderson, 1983).

LIFESTYLE/ADAPTIVE PERFORMANCE

This model is based upon ideas that come from anthropology, economics, politics, psychology, physiology, and history. It emphasizes how a human goes about satisfying his or her needs in these various contexts. The core concepts are related to the domains of self-care, intrinsic gratification, contributing to the welfare of others, and interpersonal relationships (Fidler, 1996). Culture, a group's design for acceptable beliefs and behavior, is an important feature of this model. Achievement of the skills necessary to be successful in each domain depends on cultural norms and values; consequently, culture can affect health. This model parallels the psychodynamic and developmental theories of human behavior more closely than most other occupational therapy models.

In this model, illness is defined by the inability to perform in the domains of self-care, intrinsic gratification, social contribution, and relationships in their own environment. Feelings of helplessness and being out of control, caused either by internal or external circumstances, can result in dysfunction. The origin of illness can be biomechanical, biochemical, or environmental, but the effect is a decrease in independent need satisfaction. This perspective, which unifies theories from several disciplines, is considered to be inclusive and adaptable to eclecticism.

The view of crafts in this model relates strongly to purpose. Exercise is seen as having a single purpose—body motion—while occupations other than exercise may combine multiple purposes or meanings. *Doing* becomes a critical skill, and doing in a group is the most valuable. Through doing, clients learn culturally acceptable ways of communication as well as actual task skills (Fidler, Fidler, 1978; Fidler, 1969).

A psychological theory of human behavior that fits in some ways with the lifestyle/adaptive performance model is that of Abraham Maslow, a psychologist who focused on what people can do rather than what they cannot do. He saw human life as a hierarchical approach to satisfying human needs. Many occupational therapists use his theories, which are basically psychological approaches that are easily adapted to occupational therapy (Maslow, 1968). A more thorough explanation of this theory is found in the Introduction to Chapter 8. It includes a diagram of how crafts can be conceptualized for a hierarchy of satisfaction of human needs (see Figure 8-1).

REHABILITATION MODEL

This model has its roots in physical medicine (Neistadt, Crepeau, 1997). It considers the potential for improvement in human function. Humans have many more capabilities and resources than they ever use (Kessler, 1947). Humans are thought to have segments in their lives like physical, mental, social, and vocational (Krusen, Koftke, Ellwood, 1968; Rusk, 1971). Each of these aspects of the human is assessed and treated in an interdisciplinary approach by individual professionals. The professionals then meet as a team to share their findings and to develop a comprehensive plan with the client (Garrison, 1995). This approach was the forerunner to holistic client care (Krusen, Koftke, Ellwood, 1968).

The rehabilitation approach has been traditionally reserved for the chronically ill and disabled. Their illness or dysfunction usually results from external trauma or through endogenous illness. Problems amenable to the rehabilitation model are often problems for which there is no permanent solution or cure (Neistadt, Crepeau, 1997; Kessler, 1947; Krusen, Koftke, Ellwood, 1968; Rusk, 1971). The World Health Organization *International Classification of Impairments, Disabilities and Handicaps* (WHO, 1994) fits with this approach (Christiansen, Baum, 1997;

Garrison, 1995). The therapist-client relationship is one of teacher-learner (Neistadt, Crepeau, 1997; Garrison, 1995). Activities/occupations are chosen in this model because they challenge the client to go beyond what he or she could do or help the client reach the limit of his or her capabilities. Crafts may be used to achieve goals in physical, mental, social, or vocational spheres, but work simulation or vocational tasks predominate. The client may engage in activities of daily living (ADLs) as an adjunct to vocational roles. The current ADL approach used in many occupational therapy rehabilitation treatment settings has reduced the use of crafts as a treatment medium. Cooking is the main craft currently being used (Titus, 1997).

MODEL OF HUMAN OCCUPATION

This evolving theory is based on the General Systems Theory (Kielhofner, 1995). The Model of Human Occupation has three subsystems: the volitional subsystem, the habituation subsystem, and the mind-brain-body performance subsystem. Each subsystem is equally important; however, they have changing levels of power and importance. The volitional subsystem includes ideas about personal causation, self-knowledge, values, interests, and choices. The habituation subsystem has to do with the habits and learned roles that give a person stability so that he or she needs not think through each action required to perform. The mind-brain-body performance subsystem puts it all together for the person to perform an action or occupation. Concepts of cause and effect are important in this model, as they are related to a person's idea of his or her own capability to control what happens to him or her (Kielhofner, 1995).

This model takes an interactive approach in which context (a concept that includes environment and issues related to time in a person's life) is considered central to occupational performance. Humans are intrinsically motivated to become involved with their environments. Environmental interaction in its broadest sense is the essence of human occupation, which is occupational therapy's ultimate domain of concern. Occupation is expressed as an innate need to participate in society and culture. In this model, it is important for a client to choose his or her own activities/occupations (Early, 1993). This has importance for therapists, as they will encourage clients to choose an activity/occupation rather than assigning one.

Dysfunction is defined as the lack of meaning or purpose and a failure to explore and become involved with the environment. Illness or dysfunction is not a static condition but has different levels and changes with the environment.

Activities/occupations such as crafts used in this model provide a treatment environment. The client chooses to explore and work with materials. The treatment setting provides a variety of craft samples and materials so that the client will be motivated to explore and achieve some mastery of the craft. Competence in a craft will result from development of skill in handling the materials. Concurrently, the client learns the role of worker or crafts person, thus experiencing a feeling of mastery of the clinical environment. It is this feeling of competence or mastery that can be transferred to exploration of the environment outside the hospital (Kielhofner, 1995).

OCCUPATIONAL ADAPTATION

This model is a relative newcomer in the occupational therapy profession's stream of thinking. It first appeared in the *American Journal of Occupational Therapy* in 1992 (Neistadt, Crepeau, 1997; Christiansen, Baum, 1997; Schkade, Shultz, 1992a, 1992b). In this theory, humanity adapts to change through being occupied. It shares with the Lifestyle/Adaptive Performance Model and the Model of Human Occupation the idea of *intrinsic motivation* to do activities/occupations. The authors of this model attempt to be inclusive of several different established occupational therapy theories. It shares the idea of *mastery* with the Developmental/ Spatiotemporal Model. Taken into account in the Model of Occupational Adaptation is the unique experience of clients as they attempt to adapt to changing conditions either within themselves or in their external environments. A condition is designated as illness in this theory, when a client is unable to proceed through the process of adapting to change.

In analyzing the client, three systems are considered: psychosocial, sensorimotor, and cognitive. Studies of adaptive response by Canadian researcher Hans Selye in the 1950s influenced this occupational therapy model. This theory assumes that there is a limited amount of energy available for each client to expand on any particular adaptive response. Part of the therapist's job is to assist the clients to pace themselves so they do not exhaust their energy supply. Related to crafts, this theory would focus on the motivation the client has toward an activity/occupation. It would ask whether the craft is guiding the client toward mastery and being able to generalize what is learned to other tasks. We can expect this theory to undergo refinement as therapists use it in practice.

REFERENCES

Allen, C. K. (1985). *Occupational therapy for psychiatric diseases: Measurement and management of cognitive disabilities.* Boston: Little, Brown and Company.

Allen, C. K., Earhart, C. A., & Blue, T. (1992). *Occupational therapy treatment goals for the physically and cognitively disabled.* Rockville, MD: American Occupational Therapy Association

AOTA. *Accreditation committee accreditation manual 1991 essentials.* Rockville, MD: American Occupational Therapy Association.

Ayers, A.J. (1987). *Sensory integration and the child.* Los Angeles: Western Psychological Services.

Bonder, B. R. (1991). *Psychopathology and function.* Thorofare, NJ: SLACK Incorporated.

Bruce, M. A. G. (1994). *Cognitive rehabilitation: Intelligence, insight, and knowledge. AOTA self-study series: Cognitive rehabilitation.* Rockville, MD: American Occupational Therapy Association.

Carr, J. H,, Shepherd, R. B., Gordon, J., Gentile, A. M., Held, J. M. (1987). *Movement science: Foundations for physical therapy in rehabilitation.* Rockville, MD: Aspen Publishers, Inc.

Case-Smith, J. Allen, A. S., & Pratt, P. N. (1996). *Occupational therapy for children.* St. Louis: Mosby.

Christiansen, C., & Baum, C. (eds.). (1997). *Occupational therapy: Enabling function and well-being* (2nd ed.). Thorofare, NJ: SLACK Incorporated.

Cohen, H. (ed.). (1993). *Neuroscience for rehabilitation.* Philadelphia: Lippincott.

Duncome, L. W., Howe, M. C., & Schwartzberg, S. L. (1988). *Case simulations in psychosocial occupational therapy.* Philadelphia: F. A. Davis.

Earhart, C. A., & Allen, C. K. (1988). *Cognitive disabilities: Expanded activity analysis.* Pasadena, CA: Catherine A. Earhart.

Earhart, C. A., Allen, C. K., & Blue, T. (1993). *Allen diagnostic module.* Colchester, CT: S & S Worldwide.

Early, M. B. (1993). *Mental health concepts and techniques for the occupational therapy assistant* (2nd ed.). New York: Raven Press.

Eggers, O. (1984). *Occupational therapy in the treatment of adult hemiplegia.* Rockville, MD: Aspen Systems Corporation.

Fidler, G. S. (1969). The task-oriented group as a context for treatment. *Am J Occup Ther, 23*(1), 43-48.

Fidler, G., & Fidler, J. (1978). Doing and becoming: Purposeful action and self-actualization. *Am J Occup Ther, 32*(5), 305-310.

Fisher, A. G., Murray, E. A.. & Bundy A. C. (1991). *Sensory integration: Theory and practice.* Philadelphia, F. A. Davis Company.

Fidler, G. (1996). Lifestyle performance: From profile to conceptual model. *Am J Occup Ther, 50*(2), 139-147.

Garrison, S. J. (ed.). (1995). *Handbook of physical medicine and rehabilitation basics.* Philadelphia: Lippincott.

Gilfoyle, E. M., Grady, A. P., & Moore, J. (1990). *Children adapt* (2nd ed.). Thorofare, NJ: SLACK Incorporated.

Katz, N. (1992). *Cognitive rehabilitation: Models for intervention in occupational therapy.* Boston: Andover Medical Publishers.

Kessler, H. H. (1947). *Rehabilitation of the physically handicapped.* New York: Columbia University Press.

Kielhofner. G. (1995). *A model of human occupation: Theory and application* (2nd ed.). Baltimore: Williams & Wilkins.

Kielhofner, G. (1997). *Conceptual foundations of occupational therapy* (2nd ed.). Philadelphia: F. A. Davis.

Kramer, P., & Hinojosa, J. (1993). *Frames of reference for pediatric occupational Therapy.* Baltimore: Williams & Wilkins.

Krusen, F. H., Koftke, F. J., & Ellwood, P. M. (1968). *Handbook of physical medicine and rehabilitation.* Philadelphia: W. B. Saunders.

Llorens, L. A. (1984). Theoretical conceptualizations of occupational therapy. *Occupational therapy in mental health, 1960-1982,*1-14.

Maslow, A. (1968). *Toward a psychology of being* (Rev. ed.). New York: Van Nostrand.

Montgomery, P. C., & Connolly, B. H. (eds.). (1991). *Motor control and physical therapy: Theoretical framework and practical applications.* Hixson, TN: Chattanooga Group, Inc.

Neistadt, M. E., & Crepeau, M. B. (1997). *Willard and Spackman: Occupational therapy* (9th ed.). Philadelphia: Lippincott.

Radomski, M. V., Dougherty, P. M., Fine, S. B. & Baum, C. (1994). *Case studies in cognitive rehabilitation. AOTA self-study series: Cognitive rehabilitation.* Rockville, MD: American Occupational Therapy Association.

Reed, K. L. (1984). *Models of practice in occupational therapy.* Baltimore: Williams & Wilkins.

Reed, K. L. & Sanderson, S. R. (1983). *Concepts of occupational therapy* (2nd ed.). Baltimore: Williams & Wilkins.

Rusk, H. A. (1971). *Rehabilitation medicine* (3rd ed.). St. Louis: Mosby.

Schkade J. K. & Shultz, S. (1992a). Occupational adaptation: toward a holistic approach for contemporary practice, Part 1. *Am J Occup Ther, 46*(9), 829-837.

Schkade J. K. & Shultz, S. (1992b). Occupational adaptation: toward a holistic approach for contemporary practice, Part 2. *Am J Occup Ther, 46*(9), 829-837.

Titus, J. (1997). Treatment interventions used on level II occupational therapy fieldwork. Unpublished manuscript.

Trombly, C. A. (ed.). (1995). *Occupational therapy for physical dysfunction* (4th ed.). Baltimore: Williams & Wilkins.

Umphred, D. A. (ed.). (1995). *Neurological rehabilitation* (3rd ed.). St. Louis: Mosby.

Van Deusen, J. A. (1993). *Body image and perceptual dysfunction in adults.* Philadelphia: W. B. Saunders.

World Health Organization. (1994). *International classification or impairments, disabilities and handicaps* (10th rev. ed.). Geneva: World Health Organization.

Zemke, R. (1994). *Task skills, problem solving, and social interaction. AOTA self-study series: Cognitive rehabilitation.* Rockville, MD: American Occupational Therapy Association.

RATIONALE FOR CHOOSING AN ACTIVITY/OCCUPATION

The occupational therapy process, like the process in many other health care fields, such as nursing and physical therapy, has several steps: screening and evaluation, treatment planning, implementation of treatment, and re-evaluation (Christiansen, Baum, 1997). Some say discharge planning is a last step, however, this step can logically be included in the overall team treatment plan. Choosing an occupation/activity for a client initially occurs during the treatment planning stage.

Treatment planning logically follows evaluation since a therapist cannot make decisions about appropriate treatment until a client's functional level has been determined. A common approach to treatment planning is to list the client's problems, prioritize the problems, and compose long-term goals for the most important and/or treatable problems. Long-term goals are often thought of as the outcome the therapist and client would expect to see in 3 months to 1 year. The client and therapist together establish the goals to be included in the treatment plan (Kettenbach, 1995). For each long-term goal, the therapist, with the client, then decides on a short-term objective that could reasonably be achieved in 1 week. The last step in treatment planning is usually to list activities/occupations that could help the client accomplish the short-term objective and consequently take steps in the direction of achieving long-term goals. Sometimes there is an additional step included in treatment plans called *rationale*. Rationale is the reasoning behind the choice of particular activities/occupations. Another name for rationale is *clinical reasoning* (Christiansen, Baum, 1997; Neistadt, Crepeau, 1998; Sabonis-Chafee, Hussey, 1998).

Occupation, from which the profession of occupational therapy gets its name (Kielhofner, 1997), had been used interchangeably with the word *activity* until the 1980s (Nelson, 1996). The main distinction that people express when distinguishing occupations from activities is that occupations have meaning to the client, who has expectations for the final result. This implies that the meaning for the term *occupation* is synonymous with the term *purposeful activity*, which has been used for several decades to define the core of the profession (Christiansen, Baum, 1997). At this time, many therapists use either word to designate what the client does in occupational therapy. Consequently, both terms are included here to make it easier for therapists not to be distracted by terminology they are unaccustomed to.

The following list of 21 questions is intended to be used as a guideline to assist the therapist in clinical reasoning (i.e., in developing a rationale for using a particular occupation/activity with a particular client).

QUESTIONS FOR
GUIDING CLINICAL REASONING

1. Which of the client's goals/objectives can be achieved by doing this occupation/activity?
2. What clients have you had in the past with similar problems? What activities/occupations did you use with them?
3. What occupation/activity would the client like to do? Are the client's reasons for choosing that activity logical and reasonable to you?
4. What occupation/activity can you reasonably expect the client to accomplish in the time you expect to work with him or her?
5. Could this occupation/activity help change the client's habits?
6. What occupation/activity can help the client learn new skills?
7. What occupation/activity could have an effect on the client's underlying disease process?
8. What occupation/activity would allow the client to use his or her remaining capabilities?
9. What occupation/activity would make use of the client's remaining strengths?
10. Will the client's disability require that the therapist do part of the occupation/activity for him or her?
11. What occupations/activities fit the client's cultural identity?
12. What occupations/activities fit the person's age and sexual identity?
13. What factors in this occupation/activity could make the client worse rather than better?
14. Can the occupation/activity be completed before the client is discharged?

15. Is the client physically, emotionally, and cognitively able to complete the occupation/activity?
16. Do you have the materials to perform the occupation/activity or can they reasonably be obtained?
17. How easy would it be to make this occupation/activity more challenging or less demanding for the client?
18. If you were called away before the client completed the occupation/activity, could another therapist easily take over?
19. Is this occupation/activity appropriate for the theoretic model you are using?
20. How can you measure the client's progress toward the goal for which the occupation/activity was chosen?
21. How will you know that the goal of this occupation/activity has been achieved?

In summary, this list of questions attempts to guide the student or beginning therapist through the thought process that seasoned therapist often do instantly and without apparent effort. That effortless quality usually follows frequent use of the clinical thinking process. Developing a rationale for the chosen occupation/activity can give the therapist confidence, which indeed contributes to healing (Christiansen, Baum, 1997; Neistadt, Crepeau, 1998).

REFERENCES

Christiansen, C., & Baum, C. (1997). *Occupational therapy: Enabling function and well-being* (2nd ed.). Thorofare, NJ: SLACK Incorporated.
Kettenbach, G. (1995). *Writing soap notes* (2nd ed.). Philadelphia: F. A. Davis.
Kielhofner, G. (1997). *Conceptual foundations of occupational therapy* (2nd ed.). Philadelphia: F. A. Davis.
Neistadt, M. E., & Crepeau, E. B. (eds.). (1998). *Willard & Spackman's occupational therapy* (9th ed.). Philadelphia: Lippincott.
Nelson, D. N. (1996). Therapeutic occupation: A definition. *Am J Occup Ther, 50*(10), 775-782.
Sabonis-Chafee, B., & Hussey, S. M., (1998). *Introduction to occupational therapy* (2nd ed.). St. Louis: Mosby.

UNIFORM TERMINOLOGY AND CRAFTS

The first time the American Occupational Therapy Association formalized uniform terminology was in 1979 (AOTA, 1979). A decade later, it was rewritten and published in the *American Journal of Occupational Therapy Uniform Terminology for Occupational Therapy*, Second Edition (1989a, 1989b). Only 5 years later, a third document was adopted (AOTA, 1994). Each effort to document the special language of occupational therapy has refined and refocused our practice. The third document has three foci of concern: performance areas, performance components, and performance contexts.

Performance areas (Table 4-1) include self-care occupations, which are sometimes called *activities of daily living*. However, performance areas include much more than dressing, grooming, toileting, and feeding. They also include important ways in which humans care for themselves, such as health maintenance and medication routines, socialization and communication, mobility at home and in the community, response to emergencies, and sexual expression.

Other performance areas are work-like and play/leisure activities/occupations. Many craft activities fall into these two categories. Traditionally, craftwork was considered to be skilled labor or work for employment. Because it is difficult to support oneself on the earnings from craftwork in the Information Age, such activities/occupations are now considered leisure or play except by artists and artisans. Consequently, in using the uniform terminology document to think about crafts, these particular areas of human need, play, and work will be the areas of concentration.

I. Performance Areas	II. Performance Component	III. Performance Contexts
A. Activities of Daily Living	A. Sensorimotor Component	A. Temporal Aspects
1. Grooming	1. Sensory	1. Chronological
2. Oral Hygiene	a. Sensory Awareness	2. Developmental
3. Bathing/Showering	b. Sensory Processing	3. Life Cycle
4. Toilet Hygiene	(1) Tactile	4. Disability Status
5. Personal Device care	(2) Proprioceptive	B. Environment
6. Dressing	(3) Vestibular	1. Physical
7. Feeding and Eating	(4) Visual	2. Social
8. Medication Routine	(5) Auditory	3. Cultural
9. Health Maintenance	(6) Gustatory	
10. Socialization	(7) Olfactory	
11. Functional Communication	c. Perceptual Processing	
12. Functional Mobility	(1) Stereognosis	
13. Community Mobility	(2) Kinesthesia	
14. Emergency Response	(3) Pain Response	
15. Sexual Expression	(4) Body Scheme	
B. Work and Productive Activities	(5) Right-Left	
1. Home Management	Discrimination	
a. Clothing Care	(6) Form Constancy	
b. Cleaning	(7) Position in Space	
c. Meal Preparation/Cleanup	(8) Visual-Closure	
d. Shopping	(9) Figure Ground	
e. Money Management	(10) Depth Perception	
f. Household Maintenance	(11) Spatial Relations	
g. Safety Procedures	(12) Topographical	
2. Care of Others	Orientation	
3. Educational Activities	2. Neuromusculoskeletal	
4. Vocational Activities	a. Reflex	
a. Vocational Exploration	b. Range of Motion	
b. Job Acquisition	c. Muscle Tone	
c. Work or Job Performance	d. Strength	
d. Retirement Planning	e. Endurance	
e. Volunteer Participation	f. Postural Control	
C. Play or Leisure Activities	g. Soft Tissue Integrity	
1. Play or Leisure Exploration	3. Motor	
2. Play or Leisure Performance	a. Gross Coordination	
	b. Crossing the Midline	
	c. Laterality	
	d. Bilateral Integration	
	e. Motor Control	
	f. Praxis	
	g. Fine Coordination/Dexterity	
	h. Visual-Motor Integration	
	i. Oral-Motor Control	
	B. Cognitive Integration and Cognitive Components	
	1. Level of Arousal	
	2. Orientation	
	3. Recognition	
	4. Attention Span	
	5. Initiation of Activity	
	6. Termination of Activity	
	7. Memory	
	8. Sequencing	
	9. Categorization	
	10. Concept Formation	
	11. Spatial Operations	
	12. Problem Solving	
	13. Learning	
	14. Generalization	
	C. Psychosocial Skills and Psychological Components	
	1. Psychological	
	a. Values	
	b. Interests	
	c. Self-Concept	
	2. Social	
	a. Role Performance	
	b. Social Conduct	
	c. Interpersonal Skills	
	d. Self-Expression	
	3. Self-Management	
	a. Coping Skills	
	b. Time-Management	
	c. Self-Control	

Table 4-1.

Uniform Terminology for Occupational Therapy. Reprinted with permission from the American Occupational Therapy Association.

Performance components (see Table 4-1) are the various specific functions within the domains of sensorimotor responses and behaviors, cognition, psychosocial capabilities, and other psychological functions. Each of these may be important in occupational performance of a task. These categories of performance components have a number of items included within them.

Performance context is the new aspect of human function included in the 1994 version of *Uniform Terminology*. The dictionary defines context as the "setting in which something occurs" (Morehead, Morehead, 1995). In occupational therapy terms, this means time in a person's life, disability status, and condition of health, as well as environmental and socio-cultural forces. Performance context encourages the therapist to look at all aspects of the life of the client.

If a therapist uses uniform terminology as a guideline rather than a boundary limiting practice, it can ease the process of documenting treatment plans and outcomes. It is possible to use uniform terminology as a fence to say, "This is where my responsibilities end with a client." Because occupational therapists are always expected to view the client in a holistic way, it is important not to have the mindset of limiting the possible ways of working with a client. Nonetheless, uniform terminology, carefully observed, does structure craft use in the clinic.

PHYSICAL DISABILITIES

If the reader thinks of a male European-American stroke patient with mild non-dominant hemiparesis who would like to continue a craft of fly tying started in the inpatient clinic, what performance components might come up? Initially, the performance areas would be considered. Fly tying for this man would be a *play* or *leisure activity* because it is associated with his long-time hobby of fly fishing. The performance components that a therapist might consider in making a treatment plan would include tactile and visual. In the category of *sensory processing*, one would consider stereognosis, kinesthesia, pain response, and right-left discrimination in the category of *neuromusculoskeletal*; motor control, praxis, fine motor coordination/dexterity, and visual-motor integration in the *motor* category; memory, sequencing, and spatial operations in the *cognitive* category; interests, and role performance in the *psychosocial* category.

The performance contexts for this man would include his home, in which he is having his home health occupational therapy treatment; his age, which is 63; his developmental stage, which would be as a grandparent and his disability status and the manual activity disabilities,[6] which would allow him to continue this previously learned task. The cultural value European-American males place on fishing is one of a masculine activity. In choosing assessments for this client to see if he is capable of fly tying, the therapist would choose assessments that address these performance areas, components, and contexts of his life.

PEDIATRICS

Another example might be a child of mixed racial background who lives in a developmental center and is learning to hold scissors in order to prepare to participate in the facility's classroom education program. The inability to successfully hold the scissors interferes with the performance areas of work and productive activities (specifically safety procedures), as well as educational activities, vocational activities (specifically work or job performance), play, and leisure activities.

Performance components that might be considered for intervention to assist this future student might be sensory processing, such as tactile and visual; perceptual processing, such as kinesthesia, right-left discrimination, visual closure, and figure ground; neuromusculoskeletal, such as muscle tone, postural control, motor control, praxis, fine coordination/dexterity, and visual-motor integration; cognitive integration such as recognition, initiating and terminating an activity, sequencing spatial operations, and problem solving; and psychosocial skills and psychological components, such as self-control.

Performance contexts for this future student might include her age, level of her development mentally, emotionally, and physically, and how disabled she is. It might also include where the intervention takes place, including the toys and furniture present, as well as which people will be present at the time of treatment and in follow-up care. The cultural background of this future student as well as her care givers' is important. The culture of the developmental center is also an important factor. Health care facilities develop their own culture over time. The culture of the center would include the ethnic cultures of the people that staff it, administrative policies related to clothing and behavior, which other health care professionals work there, and the culture of the surrounding community.

In this case, many of the nursing assistants are African-Americans. Their wages are low and the culture does not emphasize providing children in their community with arts and crafts materials at home. Consequently, in considering the cultural performance context, the therapist would recognize that it might be unrealistic to expect these nursing assistants to provide experiences for this future student that they do not provide for their own children. This would mean that if the therapist wants the child to have carry-over from the treatment session, the therapist would have to supplement the context by educating the nursing assistants about the need for the child to practice cutting with scissors.

MENTAL HEALTH

Another example of using uniform terminology in thinking about craft use with a client would be the case of a 20-year-old European-American male recently diagnosed as schizophrenic. In a community mental health center outpatient program, the client decided to make a wooden toy for his son, who lives with the client's girlfriend and is the child's mother.

The performance areas involved in the endeavor are care of others and play or leisure activities/occupations. He is trying to learn parenting skills so he can be supportive of his girlfriend, who is the child's main caretaker. Making this toy assists him in concentrating on this area of family life.

The performance components important to his successful completion of this task are the sensory processing components of tactile, proprioceptive, and visual sensations; perceptual processing components of kinesthesia, pain response, right-left discrimination, form constancy, visual-closure, figure ground, and depth perception (which are distortions of perception (WHO, 1980); neuromusculoskeletal components of range of motion, muscle tone, strength, endurance, postural control, and postural alignment; motor components of gross coordination, crossing the midline, bilateral integration, motor control, praxis, fine coordination/dexterity, and visual-motor integration; cognitive components of attention span, memory, sequencing, spatial operations, problem solving, initiation, and termination of an activity; psychosocial components of interest, self-expression, and self-management.

The performance contexts that would be involved in woodworking for this client are the occupational work space, the tools required, the fact that the client is a parent at such a young age, his perceptual difficulties resulting from schizophrenia, and his Irish-German-American background and cultural expectations for capability of men to be able perform woodwork.

GERIATRICS

A Scotch/Irish-American female client in a geropsychiatric inpatient unit could benefit by the therapist's use of uniform terminology in guiding the occupational therapy approach to assessment, writing goals, and choosing craft activity/occupations with her. This 78-year-old retired, widowed, rural homemaker, who lives in an assisted living facility, is experiencing short-term memory problems that frighten her and exasperate her caregivers. She wants to work on quilts, as she has done throughout her life.

The performance areas involved in such a craft activity include socialization, safety procedures, work or job performance, and play/leisure activities. In her past as a farmer's wife, she had used quilting as a way to salvage old clothing and save money on bedding, thus qualifying it as a work activity/occupation since it was part of the farm economy. Now in the assisted living residence, she joins a quilting group, which functions as a leisure activity and socialization opportunity.

The performance components that are affected by her memory problem are primarily cognitive. Her attention span, initiation and termination of activity, memory, sequencing, and problem solving are affected. She is able to perform the actual quilting due to years of habituation of the movements required for the task. The memory problem she experiences is in how to plan to cut out the pattern and piece it together. The psychosocial components of her values and interests in quilting are important motivators.

The performance contexts that are important relating to quilting for this women are that this occupation has been part of each of her cycles of life. She is able to do the activity/occupation despite her cognitive disability (WHO, 1980). The environment of the facility, the social opportunities of an arranged program for residents, and her Scotch-Irish cultural heritage are contextual factors to be considered in choosing quilting.

TREATMENT PLANNING

One method of using uniform terminology to guide treatment interventions is to use the list of the uniform terminology outline to select appropriate problems upon which to focus. In thinking about goals, the therapist might use the performance areas to guide vocabulary choice in formulating the long-term goals and performance components to more specifically focus on what can be accomplished in a short time. Performance contexts will assist the therapist in providing a rationale consistent with the client's life situation.

SUMMARY

The uniform terminology document of the American Occupational Therapy Association makes logical sense in moving from a more global view of a client's disability problems toward the specific activities that can provide steps toward solving problems. It is important for the therapist to use it to simplify the treatment planning process rather than to limit the scope of practice.

REFERENCES

American Occupational Therapy Association. (1979). *Occupational therapy product output reporting system and uniform terminology for reporting Occupational therapy services.* Rockville, MD: American Occupational Therapy Association.
American Occupational Therapy Association. (1989). Uniform Terminology for Occupational Therapy (2nd ed.). *Am J Occup Ther, 43*(12), 808-815.
American Occupational Therapy Association. (1994). Uniform terminology for occupational therapy (3rd ed.). *Am J Occup Ther, 48*(11), 1047-1054.
American Occupational Therapy Association. (1994). Uniform terminology (3rd ed.): application to practice. *Am J Occup Ther, 48*(11), 1055-1059.
Morehead, A., & Morehead, L. (eds.). (1995). *The New American Webster Handy College Dictionary* (3rd ed.). New York: Signet.
World Health Organization. (1980). *International Classification of Impairments, Disabilities, and Handicaps,* Geneva, Switzerland: World Health Organization.

ANALYZING AND GRADING ACTIVITIES

ANALYSIS ACTIVITY

Occupational therapy is a "doing" profession. Clients are involved in doing activities/occupations. While the term *activity analysis* is one that all therapists recognize, as the profession of occupational therapy struggles to define the word *occupation*, it is important to have a definition of occupation to differentiate it from *activity*. Dictionary definitions are usually understood by people outside the profession; consequently, they are presented before the elaboration that occupational therapy has provided for these terms.

Activity: state of being active (Christiansen, Baum, 1997); a function; event (Morehead, Morehead, 1995).
Occupation: means of filling one's time; regular employment; a job (Christiansen, Baum, 1997).

Occupational therapists interpret these dictionary definitions to imply that activities differ from occupations in that they are not required to have meaning or a definable outcome. Occupations, on the other hand, imply that the individual involved in an occupation is an active, rather than passive, participant; what is being done is meaningful to the person, and there is a goal to be accomplished (Morehead, Morehead, 1995). Nonetheless, there is an expectation in occupational therapy of participation that can be either active or passive. A passive activity might be one in which a client simply attends a group but is not active in the group occupational therapy. Clients are seldom done unto, as are many clients treated by other professions. Treatment in occupational therapy involves doing something. Consequently, there is a need to be skilled in analysis of what a person must do in each activity/occupation used with clients.

Over the years, occupational therapists have developed their own vocabulary to describe what they do. This has been, and continues to be, codified into a language called uniform terminology, as described in the previous chapter. The activity analysis presented and described in this chapter is based upon the 1994 *Uniform Terminology* (AOTA, 1994). It can be used with any of the theoretical models described in Chapter 2.

In the 1940s, when there was a great deal of emphasis on physical dysfunction following World War II, the term activity analysis developed as a descriptive phrase for what a therapist must go through to understand what motions normally occur in different craft activities/occupations. The phrase activity analysis began to be used in texts written by American occupational therapists (Willard, Spackman, 1947) but not by British occupational therapists (Colson, 1944; Haworth, MacDonald, 1946). While the concept of considering all aspects of an activity/occupation—psychological, physical, social, and economic—was gradually gaining acceptance, the phrase activity analysis was not used consistently until the 1960s (Council on Physical Medicine of the American Medical Association, 1947; Department of the Army, 1951; Fidler, Fidler, 1963; MacDonald, 1960; Scullen, 1956; Willard, Spackman, 1963). During the 1980s, Barris, Cordero, and Christiaansen emphasized, "that it is more important to know how to analyze and modify activities than it is to know how to do these activities oneself" (1986). Realistically, one cannot analyze an activity/occupation one does not know how to do.

Many different methods of activity/occupational analysis have been developed since 1960. As practice issues have evolved over the decades, as the emphasis changed from physical to emotional and back to physical, and as specialties in practice emerged, different analyses developed for each specialty. Within the specializations in occupational therapy, each activity analysis has a slightly different organizational emphasis and asks for slightly different information. The trend toward holism, however, was reflected in 1988 with the development of one integrated activity analysis form (Hopkins, Smith, 1988). Some newer texts completely ignore the term activity analysis (Morehead, Morehead, 1995; Christiansen, Baum, 1991), while others present activity analysis but do not provide an outline of what is included (Sarbonis-Chafee, Hussey, 1998). This term was central to occupational therapy treatment for 50 years, and though it appears to be receiving less emphasis now, that does not diminish the necessity to go through this process in calculating the requirements and benefits that a task may have for a client.

An activity/occupational analysis theoretically cannot exist without a client in mind; consequently, the activity/occupational analysis given in this text requires that the therapist use a hypothetical client in critically examining the requirements to do a task.

The sample blank activity/occupation analysis form (Form 5-1) was developed for crafts and activities presented in this book. It uses the same vocabulary as uniform terminology, though arranged in a way to sequentially take the user of this form through factors to be considered. It is not necessarily in the same order as the uniform terminology (see Table 4-1). For example, the performance contexts are at the beginning of the activity analysis form because they guide the user to look first at the global world of the client rather than looking at smaller pieces of the client's needs and capabilities, or the craft's individual requirements. If the uniform terminology terms do not apply to craftwork, they are not included.

While the form is intended to be holistic in its approach, which means "all aspects of a client's health" (Christiansen, Baum, 1997), it breaks down the performance contexts, performance areas, and performance components, which requires the user to fill in the appropriate information. To break something apart is the antithesis of holistic. However, for the analytic efficiency required in the modern health care system, this form allows therapists to use only what is necessary for each individual client. It is possible to use the form to focus on only one performance area, or subset of performance components, if that is all that the craft requires or the client needs. To use the form in this fashion, the therapist would complete Parts I through XI and then complete the appropriate performance component sections. The therapist is encouraged to fill in all the information called for after each word or phrase. If the information asked for is not applicable to the craft activity, the therapist should write "N/A" (not applicable) in that space. A completed version of this sample activity/occupation analysis form is located in Appendix III.

GRADING

Crafts can offer satisfaction at almost any functional level by either increasing or decreasing their complexity or size. By approaching each craft with a view of changing its level of difficulty, a therapist can match an activity/occupation with the treatment needs of the full spectrum of clients. Grading, as used by occupational therapists, may be defined by Webster's (1969) definition of gradual, which comes from the same root word:

Gradual: adj. 1. proceeding by steps or degrees; 2. moving, changing, or developing by fine, slight, or often imperceptible degrees.

Many clients improve, while others deteriorate. A craft that the client may have accomplished or been proficient in at an earlier period may still be simplified.

This is central to occupational therapy—to match or adapt the activity to the client. By approaching each craft with the sure knowledge that it can be made simpler or more complex according to the needs of the clients, the therapist can be confident that a client is allowed to choose a craft that fits his or her self-concept.

Form 5-1.
Basic Form

   I. Name of activity/occupation
  II. Performance contexts (for a hypothetical client)
     A. Client's age/gender
     B. Diagnosis/disability status
     C. Residential environment
     D. Family/friends situation
     E. Ethnic/cultural identification
     F. Economic/employment status
     G. Educational level
     H. Treatment setting
       1. Size of room
       2. Working space per person
       3. Furniture arrangement (use diagram if necessary)
       4. Lighting
       5. Equipment and appliances
       6. Ventilation and temperature
 III. Treatment goal for which activity/occupation is intended
 IV. Materials and tools needed; amount and cost of each
  V. Pre-session preparation
     A. By whom (aide, assistant, client)
     B. Steps in preparation
     C. Time required
 VI. Placement of tools and materials (i.e., in cupboard, on table)
VII. Steps in craft activity (number in order and describe each step, including time required)
VIII. Method of instruction (i.e., demonstration, verbal directions, audio or visual aid)
 IX. Opportunities for grading activity
     A. Simpler to more complex
     B. Complex to simpler
  X. Precautions (i.e., balance/gait or suicidal risk)
 XI. Performance areas—Into which does this craft activity/occupation fall and why?
     A. Health maintenance
     B. Home management
     C. Care of others
     D. Educational level (use either age or grade-level performance expectations)
     E. Vocational/retirement (opportunities for practicing work-related skills)
       1. Taking instruction
       2. Accepting authority

Form 5-1.
Basic Form, continued

3. Being able to adapt
4. Setting goals
5. Planning and performing independently/cooperatively
6. Practicing stress-management skills
7. Demonstrating good body mechanics
8. Timing/waiting
9. Counting
10. Making decisions
11. Self evaluation

F. Play/leisure exploration
G. Play/leisure performance

XII. Performance components
   A. Sensorimotor
     1. Sensory/awareness processing
       a. Does the skin receive temperature and pressure stimulation during this craft?
       b. Is it essential to feel the relationship of body parts to each other for performance of this activity? (i.e., holding with one hand while pushing with the palm of the other)
       c. Does the activity require that the client be able to distinguish the position and movement of the head during this activity? (i.e., bending over)
       d. Does the craft stimulate the visual system? How?
       e. Is the auditory system stimulated by this craft? How?
       f. Does the gustatory system receive stimulation? How?
       g. Does the craft stimulate the olfactory system? How?
     2. Perceptual processing
       a. Is stereognosis, knowing by feel, necessary during this process? When?
       b. It is necessary to be able to distinguish joint movement? Which joints?
       c. Does this craft cause any negative sensations? (i.e., pain, bad smells)
       d. Is awareness of body scheme or position of the body in space essential in this activity/occupation? When?
       e. Does the client need to discriminate the right from left side in this craft? When?
       f. Is it necessary to discriminate whether forms, shapes, and spaces are the same? When?
       g. Will it be necessary to identify an incomplete object or picture in order to know how to complete the craft?

Form 5-1.
Basic Form, continued

(i.e., understand sequential diagrams in craft instrutions)

    h. Will it be necessary for the client to distinguish a figure or object from its background?

    i. Will the client be required to use depth perception to perform this task? Explain.

    j. Is it necessary to distinguish the position of objects in relation to each other and/or to move from one object to another? Explain.

B. Neuromusculoskeletal

    1. Could craft activity stimulate a reflexive movement? (i.e., loud noise causing the client to jump)

    2. Which joint movements are involved? (i.e., flexion, extension, abduction, adduction)

    3. Are movements passive or active?

    4. How much range-of-motion is necessary? (i.e., full, limited, moderate)

    5. Is muscle tone limiting completion of the task? i.e., spasticity, flaccidity)

    6. How will the client be positioned? (i.e., seated, standing, lying down)

    7. How much endurance (time) and strength (muscle power) are required in each position?

    8. Does the client need to be able to maintain upright posture?

C. Motor

    1. Which muscle groups are involved?

    2. Is it necessary to move the eyes or limbs across the mid-sagital line of the body?

    3. Must both sides of the body work together?

    4. Does the craft require planning ahead before moving?

    5. Is fine motor control or finger dexterity required?

    6. Must visual information be coordinated with body movement?

D. Cognition

    1. Orientation (Is each of the below necessary? Why?)

        a. Time

        b. Place

        c. Person

    2. Recognition (able to identify things previously presented)

    3. Memory

        a. Short-term memory requirements (10 seconds to 10 minutes)

Form 5-1.
Basic Form, continued

b. Recent memory requirements (hours, days, months)

c. Long-term memory requirements (years to remote past)

4. Attention span; longest period of time required for concentration on one step

5. Initiating and terminating an activity appropriately

6. Sequencing actions in the correct order

7. Mentally manipulating objects spatially

8. Problem solving

a. Recognize existence of a problem

b. Think of a solution

c. Implement and evaluate the solution

9. Can the client use elsewhere what is learned in doing this craft?

E. Psychosocial

1. Does the craft provide the opportunity to discover what is valuable to the client?

2. Is the client interested enough to pay attention for the length of time required to do the craft?

3. Could the craft contribute to self-esteem? How?

4. Does the craft reinforce the client's roles and/or gender identity?

5. Is practice of social skills necessary to complete the craft? (i.e., prefacing requests with please)

6. What communication will be required?

a. By the client

b. By the therapist

c. By another client

d. With the group

7. Does the craft offer opportunities for affective expression?

a. Hostility/aggression (i.e., motions such as hammering, tearing, piercing)

b. Sadness (i.e., slow movements)

c. Happiness (i.e., pride, hope, laughter)

d. Loving (i.e., stroking, holding)

8. Does the craft provide opportunities for testing reality of the client's own perceptions/beliefs (i.e., is my behavior/perception/belief normal?)

9. What impulse control is necessary?

10. Is there an opportunity to develop leadership skills while doing the craft?

The therapist can be sure that measurable performance goals can be written and achieved for almost every craft in this text. These goals should be made with clients and discussed as a way for them to evaluate their own level of capability. This offers an opportunity to discuss how the short-term objectives of a craft project can be related to the long-term performance goals. The gradablility of crafts can be used to demonstrate the small steps clients must take to achieve true independence.

In the chapters that follow, examples of simple and more complex approaches to the same craft are included. In choosing a level of complexity, the therapist must first become proficient at activity/occupation analysis.

REFERENCES

American Occupational Therapy Association. (1994). Uniform terminology for occupational therapy (3rd ed.). *Am J Occup Ther, 48*(11), 1047-1054.

Barris, R., Cordero, J., & Christiaansen, R. (1986). Occupational therapist's use of media. *Am J Occup Ther, 40*(10), 679-684.

Christiansen, C., & Baum, C. (1991). *Occupational therapy: Overcoming human performance deficits.* Thorofare, NJ: SLACK Incorporated.

Christiansen, C., & Baum, C. (1997). *Occupational therapy: Enabling function and well-being* (2nd ed.). Thorofare, NJ: SLACK Incorporated.

Colson, J. H. C. (1944). *The rehabilitation of the injured: Occupational therapy.* London: Cassell and Company.

Council on Physical Medicine of the American Medical Association. (1947). *Manual of occupational therapy,* Chicago, IL: American Medical Association.

Department of the Army. (1951). *Occupational therapy.* Washington, DC: U.S. Government Printing Office.

Fidler, G. S., & Fidler, J. W. A. (1963). *Communication process in psychiatry: Occupational therapy.* New York: The MacMillan Co.

Haworth, N. A., MacDonald, E. M. (1946). *Theory of occupational therapy.* Baltimore: Williams & Wilkins.

Hopkins, H. L., & Smith, H. D. (1988). *Willard and Spackman's occupational therapy* (7th ed.). Philadelphia: Lippincott.

MacDonald, E. M. (1960). Occupational Therapy in Rehabilitation. London: Bailliere, Tindall and Cox.

Morehead, A., & Morehead, L. (eds.). (1995). *The new American Webster handy college dictionary* (3rd ed.). NY: Penguin Books.

Sarbonis-Chafee, B., & Hussey, S. M. (1998). *Introduction to occupational therapy* (2nd ed.). St. Louis: Mosby.

Scullen, V. (1956). *Occupational therapy manual for personnel in the New York state department of mental hygiene.* Albany, NY: State of New York Department of Mental Hygiene.

Webster's Seventh New Collegiate Dictionary. (1969). Springfield, MA: G & C Merriam Company.

Willard, H. S., & Spackman, C. S. (1947). *Principles of occupational therapy.* Philadelphia: Lippincott.

Willard, H. S., & Spackman, C. S. (1963). *Occupational therapy* (3rd ed.). Philadelphia: Lippincott.

SHALL I USE A KIT OR START FROM SCRATCH?

INTRODUCTION

If we consider *from scratch* to mean *begin by using raw materials*, occupational therapists probably never did start from scratch. In woodworking, starting from scratch would have meant cutting down the tree, aging the wood, and sawing it to proper thicknesses for use. In leathercraft, from scratch would have meant raising and killing one's own animals before tanning the hides. For needlework, the craftsperson would first need to make her own needle from bone or a quill before harvesting flax for linen or shearing the wool from sheep.

From our earliest professional writings, it is obvious that occupational therapists used materials that had some preparation before they became a part of an occupational therapy activity. Of course, there was the stray therapist who may have learned a skill such as finding and preparing her own ceramic clay, but the profession as a whole benefited from the specialization of skills that are part of the industrialized age. Consequently, the purist who asserts that occupational therapists should not use kits because they do not show clients how to start from basics is making an erroneous assumption about our past practice.

COSTS OF THERAPIST'S TIME FOR MATERIALS PREPARATION

The development and structuring of funding for providing occupational therapy treatment has radically changed our ideas about what we can and should do for our clients. Managed care pressures have limited the numbers and kinds of treatment sessions that will be reimbursed by insurance. Up until the 1970s, most occupational therapists did not worry about who was paying for treatment. They took attendance and let the financial office deal with payment for services. Little consideration was given as to whether a client had insurance or means to pay for occupational therapy. Service was provided on the basis of what the therapist perceived the client's needs to be.

By the mid 1970s, many hospitals had discovered that some insurance companies would pay an additional fee for occupational therapy over the rate charged for other daily care and treatments. This began to change the way we perceived our clients' needs. We had to document more carefully to justify to the insurance company why a client needed an hour of occupational therapy per day. We had to ask ourselves, "If this client doesn't have insurance to pay for services or even for the occupational therapy supplies, will I need to charge other clients with insurance more in order to be able to provide the needed service?" Or, "If I buy supplies of less cost and quality, will I make more money for my department?" Or, "Is my job performance to be measured by the improvement in my clients or by how much money I can make in the department?"

The answer to this last question continues to come as a shock to new therapists who entered the profession because they wanted to help people. In many situations now, when a therapist is preparing materials, it means she is not earning money for the department through chargeable client treatment. The pressure to produce revenue may cause a therapist to choose a kit rather than grading an activity up to a more complex task by using basic craft materials.

Another aspect of this issue is group versus individual treatments and the charges and costs for both. In the time before charging for treatment became such an issue, a therapist might group several clients together and work with individual clients in a less intense way but for longer periods of time. The therapist did not need to keep the time clock running in her head. As insurance companies realized that they were being charged for these new services, they began to monitor all charges more intensively. They wanted to know how the group experience was benefiting the client. In some cases, insurance companies refused to pay for group client treatment unless the client had a specific goal to improve interpersonal relations.

The guidelines for diagnostic related groups (DRGs) combined with the insurance companies' goals to monitor benefits more carefully worked to create shorter hospital stays. Clients' long-term goals, which had been emphasized, began to take a backseat to short-term objectives for occupational therapy clients. Therapists became more concerned with writing a goal that could be achieved in a week so they could document improvement in the clients' chart before they were discharged.

Because of the development of this kind of payment system, health care providers saw the need to become more accountable. This accountability affected not only charges to insurance companies, but compelled occupational therapists and occupational therapy departments to spend time in revenue-producing work that involved face-to-face contact with clients in an insurance-chargeable situation instead of doing materials preparation that could not be charged. All of these developments contributed to the profession's discomfort with the word *crafts*. Previously, we knew these crafts helped people improve their health and functional independence, but now we were being asked to tell how these results were achieved without even being allowed to use the word crafts. Crafts were just not scientific enough for a health care industry increasingly relying on evaluative testing, medication, and surgery.

As more and more people have chosen or been forced into "managed care," such things as crafts, which can maintain a client's activity/occupational level and self-esteem, are considered to be something that happens outside the health care institution. The client or his or her family must take charge and provide these activities/occupations at home or in a less costly site, such as a daycare setting rather than a hospital or clinic. Though craft involvement fits with *health maintenance*, which is one of the goals and claims of modern HMOs (health maintenance organizations), such organizations seldom credit this treatment approach with the healing capacities experienced by many clients. Anecdotal reports of benefits are discounted. Such health maintenance organizations want scientific proof that the majority of clients treated with leather craft kits showed a 50% improvement in function in a week. This proof has been difficult to provide. It is often a struggle to get such organizations to reimburse for any occupational therapy services, let alone pay for something as difficult to measure as healing results of craft work.

Space is another issue that affects whether a therapist uses kits. Storage space is not income-producing space. Formerly, when hospital stays were longer and revenue production had less emphasis, it was important to have many different craft choices available so hospitalized clients wouldn't get bored with one category of craft. Hospital stays in almost all types of treatment settings have been reduced by three quarters to one half. A much simpler inventory of craft projects is possible, requiring less storage space. Kits generally take up less space than raw materials.

USE OF AIDES AND VOLUNTEERS

Prior to the time when charging clients for services had such emphasis, registered occupational therapists often delegated materials preparation to certified occupational therapy assistants (COTA). However, COTAs' chargeable time became as important as their supervisors' time. They were revenue-producing entities. Some therapists then used aides to prepare materials because aides could not submit insurance charges. In some large institutions, aides still do some of this work.

In other institutions, volunteers are sometimes used to prepare materials for client use. Unless the volunteers have had some experience with craft materials, they require close supervision to avoid costly waste. Consequently, prepared kits are a frequently chosen alternative.

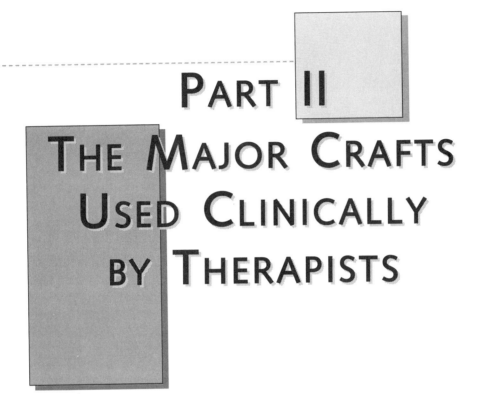

PART II
THE MAJOR CRAFTS
USED CLINICALLY
BY THERAPISTS

WOODWORKING

INTRODUCTION

Woodworking has been around for thousands of years. We have used it in dwellings and for furniture. Wood has provided some of our most basic human needs—heating and cooking, weapons, shelters, sports equipment, musical instruments, sculptures used in religious ceremonies and for decoration, and transportation such as bridges and railroad ties (Douglass, 1960; Scharff, 1952).

Woodworking encompasses a vast number of crafts: house building, boat building, furniture making, chip carving, making wood blocks for printing, whittling, toy manufacturing, wood sculpturing, and making small wooden containers for storage (*Reader's Digest*, 1979).

FREQUENCY OF USE

Approximately seven out of 10 therapists use woodcraft at some time. Cabinet making, furniture making, and other woodcrafts are commonly employed treatment methods in work-related programs (Cottrell, 1996). Wooden kits are a common project in mental health treatment.

ASSESSMENTS

Formal assessments that include woodcraft are the Work Adjustment Program (Llorens, Levy, Rubin, 1964); the Diagnostic Test Battery (Androes, Dreyfus, Bloesch, 1965); Build-a-Farm (Clark, 1978; Marmer,

1993); the Interest Checklist (Matsutsuya, 1969); the Jacobs Prevocational Skills Assessment (1991); and the Allen Diagnostic Module (Earhart, Allen, Blue, 1993). The Table of Evaluations and their Craft Components (Table 7-1) shows what other crafts may be included in each assessment. The Work Adjustment Program has three separate tasks:

- Sorting/packaging
- Assembling printed sheets
- Manufacturing objects that are made mostly of wood, such as bookshelves or furniture

The client is rated on a scale from one to six on such work skills and attitudes as attendance, motivation, dressing, and grooming. The results are helpful in vocational rehabilitation counseling (Llorens, Levy, Rubin, 1964).

In the Jacobs Prevocational Skills Assessment, there is a section called carpentry assembly. Clients are asked to name tools. They are then requested to use the tools to put in screws and hammer a nail. Their responses and actions are recorded on a checklist in relation to coordination and visual-motor, fine motor/dexterity, and cognitive performance (Jacobs, 1991).

Woodworking is the last of five subtests in the Diagnostic Test Battery. This battery may take several weeks to complete. The wood project to be assembled is a checkerboard. It includes a baseboard and a number of 2 x 2-inch squares. Some of the small wood shapes are not cut precisely. Consequently, this test involves somewhat sophisticated problem solving related to measuring the squares, counting them, and staining ones that the color does not match. The project assesses perceptual processing, cognitive skills, planning, and discrimination (Androes, Dreyfus, Bloesch, 1965).

The Build-a-Farm assessment does not formally use wood as do the previous three. Wood is included among other materials such as styrofoam, clay, and construction paper, which are presented to a small group of children or adolescents with the instruction to build a farm. This is a projective test in which the client's response to the materials is expected to reflect personality traits or psychopathology. The child's interpersonal skills are assessed by this process, in which group interactions are intrinsic in the activity (Clark, 1978; Marmer, 1993).

The Interest Checklist simply asks the clients to rate their own interest—casual, strong, or none—in 80 different activities/occupations. There are several categories that might include woodcrafts: manual arts, model building, home repairs, and woodworking. The client's responses on the checklist are then used as a basis for discussion of leisure use (Matsutsuya, 1969).

The Allen Diagnostic Module is a program for treatment and evaluation of clients. It includes 24 craft tasks, seven of which are wood assembly projects. Some of these tasks can be administered in a group setting

Table 7-1.
Evaluations and their Craft Components

	Woodworking	Leathercraft	Needlecraft	Mosaics	Ceramics	Paper Crafts	Cooking	Computer	Drawing and Painting
Allen Cognitive Levels		X							
Allen Diagnostic Module					X				X
Azima Battery					X				X
BH Battery				X					X
Bay Area Functional Performance Evaluation									X
Build-a-City						X			
Build-a-Farm	X								
Carolyn Owens Activity Battery					X				
Comprehensive Assessment Process				X		X			
Comprehensive Evaluation of Basic Living Skills							X		
Diagnostic Test Battery	X	X			X				X
Draw-a-Person									X
Fidler Activity Laboratory						X			X
Early and Advanced Switch Games								X	
Elizur Test of Psycho-Organicity									X
Goodenough-Harris Drawing Test									X
Goodman Battery					X	X			X
The Gremlin Hunt								X	
Gross Activity Battery					X				X
Homemaking Evaluation			X						
House-Tree-Person									X
Interest Checklist	X	X	X	X	X		X		X
Instrumental ADL							X		
Jacobs Prevocational Skills			X	X			X		
Kinetic Family Drawing									X
Lafayette Clinic Battery						X			
Magazine Picture Collage						X			
Mattis Dementia Rating Scale									X
Milwaukee Evaluation of Daily Living Skills			X						
Nedra Gilette Battery					X	X			
Nelson Clark's "Clay Test"						X			
O'Kane Diagnostic Battery						X			X
Perkins Tile Task					X				
Scoreable Self-Care Evaluation							X		
Shoemyen Diagnostic Battery					X	X			
Street Survival Skills Questionnaire							X		
Tiled Trivet Assessment					X				
Visual Organization								X	
Work-Adjustment Program	X								

and some need to be administered individually. Criteria are given for each task to guide the therapist in discovering at which of the six cognitive levels the client is functioning (Earhart, Allen, Blue, 1993).

WORKING WITH WOOD

In the past, adapted equipment such as the bicycle saw, treadle lathe, and treadle sander were regular features of an occupational therapy clinic. These machines are seldom seen now. Some clinics have woodworking shops that contain large power tools like the drill press, table saw, jig saw, and band saw. Many clinics use only hand tools or hand-held power tools. In the following project discussions, hand tools will be described rather than power tools since hand tools are available to almost everyone. They are also less dangerous when properly used. Most woodworking tools and supplies can be purchased at hardware stores and lumberyards in the community.

Often, occupational therapists find themselves in situations in which they need to adapt equipment for their clients. For this reason, it is important for the therapist to have some skill with carpentry tools. While more commercial adaptive equipment is available every year, therapists will inevitably work with clients for whom no commercial device seems right. The therapist will need to do what we do best—adapt—and the adaptations often require the use of woodworking tools.

Supplies for a Three-Legged Stool

A very simple kit, such as a three-legged stool, in which all the parts are precut, can be completed in two sessions (Figure 7-1). A kit like this commonly contains three legs that are each 1 inch in diameter by 7 inches long, a circle of 3/4-inch thickness of pressed wood with a hardwood veneer, and sandpaper. The round holes for setting in the legs are precut.

PROCESS

1. Sand all four pieces.
2. Finish them with paint or stain.
3. When dry, glue the legs into the inset holes.

This is a simple three-step process that does not require tools except for the sandpaper and paint brushes.

Sanding has been an important tool in the occupational therapist's treatment armamentarium for many years. In the past, there were many different designs for sanding blocks, to which sandpaper was attached with tacks or staples. There were those with handles on top, with cut-out holes for the thumb or fingers, and each was planned to place a client's hand in the desired position. Cylindrical sanding blocks had sandpaper affixed to a 12-inch length of 1 1/2- to 1 1/4-inch doweling (Figure 7-2). Such a block would be used to achieve wrist extension and flexion in all

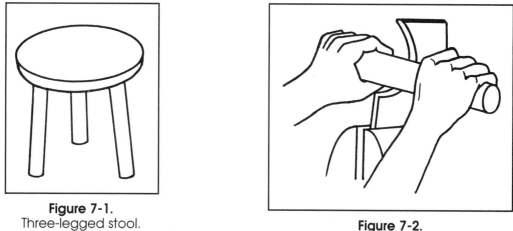

Figure 7-1.
Three-legged stool.

Figure 7-2.
Cylindrical sanding block.

finger joints. Another aid was the sanding table (Figure 7-3), which could be raised or lowered to achieve use of different upper extremity joints (Figure 7-4).

Supplies for a Pilgrim Stool

A more complicated wood project is the pilgrim stool (Figure 7-5), so called because our pilgrim ancestors designed it. This small stool has five pieces. Softwood such as pine or fir is recommended rather than a hardwood such as oak. This stool has a simple rabbet joint and is assembled with screws and wood glue.

PROCESS

1. Use a carpenter's square and pencil to transfer the enlarged pattern (Figure 7-6) from the 1-inch squared grid paper to the wood.
2. Measure and cut from a 3/4-inch board. Most of the sawing can be done with a handsaw (Figure 7-7) and coping saw (Figure 7-8).
3. Assemble the pieces to see if they fit.
4. Sand each piece.
5. Glue the pieces together.
6. Mark and drill the holes.
7. Counter sink the screw in the rabbet joint (Figure 7-9).
8. Fill the holes with wood putty and resand or cover the holes by using wood plugs made from doweling to resemble the wooden pegs used by our ancestors.
9. To finish, use stain, paint, or one of a number of waterproof finishes (Feirer, 1972).

Woodcarving

Woodcarving can be quite complicated. However, it is an often-used craft that incorporates some similar processes as chip carving.

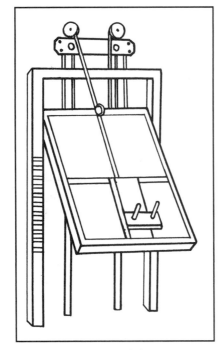

Figure 7-3.
Sanding table.

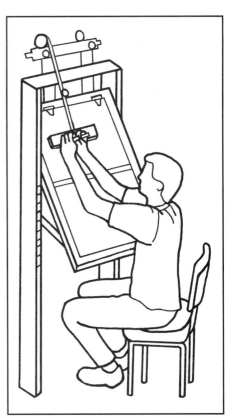

Figure 7-4.
Sanding table with the
client's shoulder in extension.

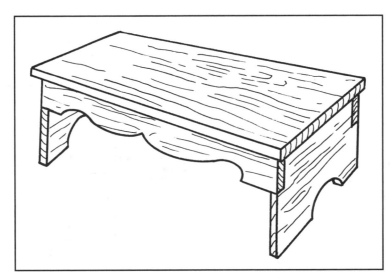

Figure 7-5.
Pilgrim stool.

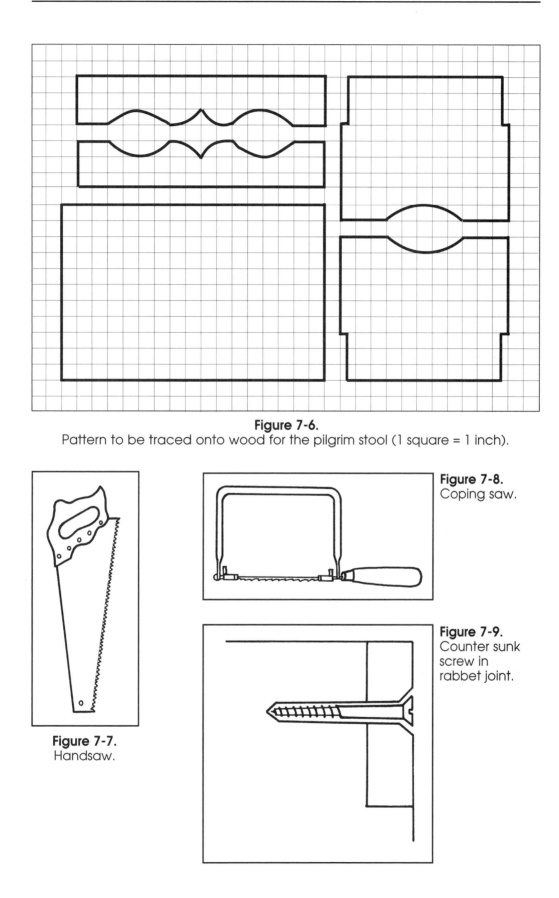

Figure 7-6.
Pattern to be traced onto wood for the pilgrim stool (1 square = 1 inch).

Figure 7-8.
Coping saw.

Figure 7-9.
Counter sunk
screw in
rabbet joint.

Figure 7-7.
Handsaw.

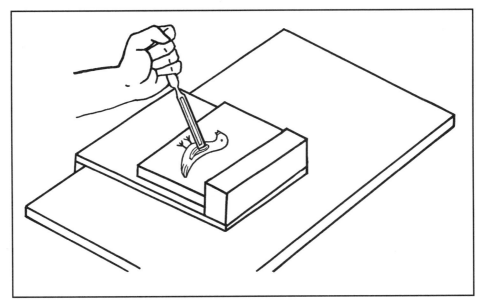

Figure 7-10.
Chip carving against a bracer board.

Woodcarving is a way of cutting a design into a wooden surface. In this way, carving can be simplified by using scraps of boards or prepared beveled wooden plaques. Balsawood, which is a very soft, light-weight wood, works well. Pine is another softwood that can be used (Marshall, 1975). Hardwood should be avoided as it is too difficult and dangerous to use in this craft. Chip carving, because of its resistive nature and because it is a constructive/destructive craft, may facilitate emotional catharsis. It requires few tools: a carving knife, a gouge, chisels, and a bracer board.

PROCESS

1. Draw the design on the flat wood with a pencil.
2. Cut the outline with a carving or utility knife (carving tools must be kept sharp by frequent honing on an oilstone)
3. Place a carving chisel in the cut outline, with the beveled edge facing the area to be chipped away. Press down and push away from the line (Figure 7-10) and remove the chip. A mallet may be used if the wood is very hard, but it is good to go slowly, as once the chip is out, it cannot be replaced.
4. Once sufficient wood has been chipped away from the outline, use a gouge with a concave-shaped blade. Start from the larger areas to be chipped away and progress to the smaller, more detailed parts. Care should be taken to keep the surface a uniform depth where wood is chipped away.
5. Sand and finish the product unless it is to be used for printing. Wood is left unfinished for printing.

MAIN THERAPEUTIC APPLICATIONS

Physical Dysfunction

Because of the traditional identification of woodworking with masculine pursuits, this can be a valuable activity/occupation for men who have lost some of their physical capacities. While large electric power tools are not discussed in this chapter, their availability and use might assist a man in compensating for lost strength. Despite the traditional association of woodworking with males, it has become more acceptable for women to do as well. Many women head single-parent families or live alone. They can attain a real sense of independence and achievement by learning basic woodworking. Home repairs, including woodworking, can be considered part of homemaking and should be included in homemaking evaluations.

Woodworking is the ideal avocational activity/occupation for the long-term client who may be living on a disability income after discharge. The expense of the large tools makes it an important consideration to help the physically disabled woodworker find a place to work. Community schools often have woodshops that students can use. Sometimes an able-bodied hobby woodcrafter may have spent considerable money to establish a workshop and yet not use it often. A disabled woodcrafter might find such a workshop to share by advertising in the local newspaper.

Range-of-motion in the hand, thumb opposition, adduction, finger flexion, and gross grasp can be achieved through carpentry. Wrist flexion, extension, and ulnar deviation can be attained with hammering and chip-carving. Flexion and extension of the elbow can be accomplished with hand drilling, sanding, hammering, and chip carving. Many shoulder movements are needed in carpentry: flexion, extension, internal rotation, external rotation, and scapular retraction. If a therapist is lucky enough to have any of the bicycle or treadle tools, much can be achieved with the lower extremities. By changing the height or position of the wood and tools, a therapist can achieve almost any joint and muscle movement. Weights can be added to increase resistance. Gravity or adaptive equipment can be used to decrease resistance. The therapist is encouraged to try each movement herself and take note of which muscles are needed (Department of the Army, 1971).

Woodworking tools can be built up with foam padding for clients with weak grip. *Note: Clients with diminished sensation, diminished circulation, or immune response need to be supervised carefully, as it is easy to scrape skin or hit a finger or thumb in woodworking.*

Mental Health

Because of their permanence, wood projects give a real feeling of accomplishment, which is associated with self-esteem. Woodworking's gradability from simple to complex provides for the wide range of functional levels found in mental health clients. This includes low-functioning mentally retarded individuals and schizophrenics to the often apparently functionally unimpaired drug addict or alcoholic. Woodworking can assess the course of deterioration or recovery in a client's condition by illustrating deficits in perceptual processing, motor control, praxis, attention span, sequencing, spatial operations, and problem solving.

While woodworking is often an individual skill and occupation, the use of small, simple precut kits allows it to be used as a group activity/occupation to enhance interpersonal skills. Clients need to share tools, glue, and containers of finish.

Pediatrics

From early childhood, toddlers enjoy hammer-and-peg toys, which help develop eye-hand coordination, motor control, and object manipulation. By the age of 3 years, many children enjoy constructing with wooden blocks. Sex role differentiation occurs around this age. The masculine identification with wood can be positive. Fathers can be encouraged to include their sons in building activities. By 4 years of age, many children envision complicated ideas but have difficulty carrying them out. Woodworking with hammer and scrap wood stimulates this kind of creativity. Normally by 5 years, a child enjoys starting something and continuing to work on it day after day. As the child begins to count and discriminate sizes and shapes, woodworking is a natural way to use numbers in measurement and comparison of shapes (Kaluger, Kaluger, 1984). Small, odd shapes and sizes of wood can be gathered at most lumber yards or cabinet-making shops. Such wood should be checked for splinters before using it with children. They like to glue these odd pieces for sculpture. Surfaces can be painted, collaged, or decoupaged.

Tongue depressors or craft sticks make nice structures. Children like to make objects that are useful. Children also like to make imaginative and symbolic objects. Some craft books include structures that may have little value or lasting interest for the child. These need to be avoided.

Woodworking from plans and drawings is too difficult for most children. They need constant one-on-one attention, which is not possible in some situations. Keep in mind, too, that in working with children, hand tools are expensive and may be underutilized in relation to their cost.

Teenagers are more likely to be able to draw and follow plans. Carved wooden sculptures will often appeal to adolescents (Gaitskell, Hurwitz, 1975).

Geriatrics

Some of the problems common to geriatric clients are diminished memory, vision, hearing, as well as increased pain. These factors affect their ability to do woodworking. Therapists can make adaptations for these problems. Precut kits often have only a few steps. The client can spend some time on one step that is repetitious, such as sanding or rubbing with stain. Each step is taught separately so that the client doesn't have to remember what comes next. When finishing an object, dark paint or stain makes it possible for the visually impaired to avoid missing any spots. There are some special precautions needed for the elderly doing woodcrafts. The hearing-impaired client may be unaware of how much noise he or she makes while hammering. Also, pain may keep a client from participating.

It is easy to injure oneself with some woodworking tools. The elderly need to have particular care taken so that they do not injure themselves, as they heal more slowly than younger people.

Clients in acute care because of a crisis situation are often not very creative. With nursing home clients, the situation lends itself to starting with very structured activities such as the three-step kit described previously, then going on to more creative projects. An elderly client who has had some furniture-building experience may enjoy miniature reproduction. Simple craft materials such as balsawood, a single-edged razor blade, and water-soluble glue can be obtained in most craft stores. Regular furniture design can be scaled down so that a weakened person can still produce fine miniature furniture (*Better Homes and Gardens*, 1966).

Elderly male clients often get very involved in woodcraft such as woodburning. Two or three elderly men doing woodburning together seem to stimulate each other to better performance. Woodburning requires minimal complex cognition but allows for much innovation. The clients may choose or draw their own designs. Older women are willing to do traditionally masculine projects like woodworking, while men are seldom willing to do feminine crafts such as needlework.

CASE STUDY

Paul, a caucasian 30-year-old sign painter who lives in a city of 35,000, became unconscious after touching a boom that was in contact with live electric wires. He was working on a scaffolding 20 feet in the air. When he became unconscious, he fell 10 feet into a tree, which broke his fall to the ground. He remained unconscious for several minutes. When he regained consciousness, some men working nearby took him to the hospital emergency department. During the week he was in the hospital, he felt groggy and in pain. The physicians were unable to find any physiological reason for his pain so they referred him to a psychiatrist.

After his discharge, he returned to work and continued to see the psychiatrist for 2 years. His relationships both at work and at home deteriorated during this time. He felt he had a good job but was afraid of losing it if he took time off for treatment of his pain. He took many medications in an attempt to rid himself of back pain. His temper became a problem, and he often got into arguments and fights with his coworkers.

At home, conflicts with his wife were about their children and her wish to return to work. They had two girls, ages 5 and 3. The 3-year-old had a diagnosis of cerebral palsy and was severely mentally retarded. She required almost total care. Now that the 5-year-old was in a kindergarten, Paul's wife wanted to return to her job as a licensed practical nurse. She had been unable to find appropriate childcare for the child with cerebral palsy. The family physician and Paul's psychiatrist favored institutionalizing the 3-year-old, but their families were opposed to the idea. Paul was suspicious of his wife wanting to return to work. He felt her desire to work was just a cover for an affair with another man. These conflicts contributed to Paul's feelings of anxiety.

A nurse in his physician's office suggested further evaluation and referred him to the outpatient unit of a rehabilitation hospital. He was evaluated by a team that included an occupational therapist, physical therapist, psychologist, and vocational evaluator. The theory of treatment used by all departments in the facility was the Rehabilitation Model. The occupational therapist gave him an interest inventory and the Minnesota Rate of Manipulation test. He checked woodworking along with photography and painting on the interest inventory as activities/occupations he enjoyed. During the Minnesota Rate of Manipulation test, he was not able to tolerate sitting through all three trials. He completed only two before his sitting tolerance and concentration gave out. Despite this, he scored high on fine and gross motor coordination. In physical therapy, he was found to be unable to walk more than one eighth of a mile. During the team meeting following the evaluations, they discussed his obvious depression.

Occupational therapy goals for Paul were to:
- Involve him in work-like activities/occupations to evaluate his future work potential
- Increase his sitting and standing tolerance and strength
- Explore his avocational interests while increasing his activity/occupational level

The therapist had Paul begin by using hand tools to make a pilgrim stool in the work-hardening program. He started slowly, taking twice as long to do each step as it normally took.

The Saturday after he had been in the program 8 weeks, he attended a craft fair with his wife. The many different kinds of woodcrafted objects that he saw stimulated him to be more creative with his woodworking in the work-hardening program. The next week, he designed and made a shelf. Several other clients liked his design so well that they asked to use it to make shelves of their own. His self-confidence and self-esteem began to increase. When the therapist wrote her progress note about him, she was able to discuss his improved self-concept.

He attempted even more difficult projects: a birdhouse, toy box for his children, dog house, and an entertainment center. As he became more involved, he did not want to attend physical therapy. The treadmill and stationary bicycle just did not motivate him like woodworking did. It was decided in a team meeting with his physician that it was time to discharge him from the rehabilitation program.

He and his wife did continue weekly visits to the psychologist for several months. Returning to his job, he found that he was able to work without pain medication. He began to use his father-in-law's garage workshop to continue doing woodcraft.

DISCUSSION QUESTIONS

1. How might it have been possible to discover Paul's interest in woodworking earlier in his treatment so that he might have gotten involved sooner?
2. What are some precautions you would need to observe with this client?
3. If this client had been a female (instead of a male) who had the same diagnosis, would this have been an appropriate craft choice? Why or why not?
4. Make a list of your own woodworking experiences. Have you included things you may have done in elementary school, Girl or Boy Scouts, 4-H Club? How could you use some of those projects with clients?

REFERENCES

Androes, L., Dreyfus, E. A., & Bloesch, M. (1965). Diagnostic test battery for occupational therapy. *Am J Occup Ther, 19*(2), 53-59.

Better Homes and Gardens. (1966). *Stitchery and Crafts.* New York: Meredith Press.

Clark, E. N. (1978). Build-a-City; Presented at 1978 American Occupational Therapy Association Conference in San Diego, California.

Cottrell, R. P. F. (1996). *Perspectives on Purposeful Activity: Foundations & Future of Occupational Therapy.* Bethesda, MD: American Occupational Therapy Association.

Department of the Army. (1971). *Craft Techniques in Occupational Therapy.* Washington, DC: U.S. Government Printing Office.

Douglass, J. H. (1960). *Woodworking with Machines.* Bloomington, IL: McKnight & McKnight Publishing Company.

Earhart, C. A., Allen, C. K., & Blue, T. (1993). *Allen Diagnostic Module: Instruction Manual.* Colchester, CT: S & S Worldwide.

Feirer, J. L. (1972). *Industrial Arts Woodworking.* Peoria, IL: Chas. A. Bennett.

Gaitskell, C. D., & Hurwitz, A. (1975). *Children and their Art* (3rd ed.). New York: Harcourt, Brace, Jovanovitch.

Jacobs, K. (1991). *Occupational Therapy: Work-Related Programs and Assessments* (2nd ed.). Boston: Little, Brown and Company.

Kaluger, G., & Kaluger, M. F. (1984). *Human Development—The Span of Life.* St. Louis: Times Mirror/Mosby College Publishing.

Llorens, L. A., Levy, R., & Rubin, E. Z. (1964). Work adjustment program. *Am J Occup Ther, 18*(1), 15-19.

Marmer, L. (1993). If you want to find out what's going on in any group, Just build a city. *Advance for Occupational Therapists, 9*(46), 12-13.

Marshall, E. M. (1975). *Occupational Therapy Fundamentals of Work.* Thorofare, NJ: SLACK Incorporated.

Matsutsuya, J. S. (1969). The interest checklist. *Am J Occup Ther, 24(4),* 323-328.

Reader's Digest. (1979). *Crafts and Hobbies.* Pleasantville, NY: The Reader's Digest Association, Inc.

Scharff, R. (1952.) *Handbook of Crafts.* Greenville, CT: Fawcett Publications.

LEATHERWORK

INTRODUCTION

It would be difficult to find a person who is not using or wearing leather or a simulation of leather: shoes, belt, hat, buttons, garments, wallets, checkcovers, notebook covers, holsters, kneepads, steering wheel covers, animal leashes, harnesses, thimbles, and balls to name just a few. Leather is our most ancient fabric (*Reader's Digest*, 1979). From archeology, we know that prehistoric humans used leather (Stohlman, Patten, Wilson, 1969). Uses of leather have been documented in a number of different cultures: Chinese, ancient Hebrew, Roman, North American Indian, Eskimo, and early European (*Reader's Digest*, 1979; Stohlman, Patten, Wilson, 1969). We do not know as much about leather as we know about ceramics because leather has been less durable over the centuries.

An important visual construct that many occupational therapists use to attempt to understand human behavior is Maslow's Hierarchy of Human Needs (Figure 8-1). It presents the idea that our basic needs control our behaviors. If your needs are physiological, they are at the survival level; if these needs are unmet, you are unable to attend to needs closer to the top of the hierarchy. Using Maslow's hierarchy, we can think in a hierarchical way about how leather was used as needs were met.

FREQUENCY OF USE

In the craft surveys, leatherwork is frequently used. Many therapists use leatherwork with their clients once per week or more; some use it

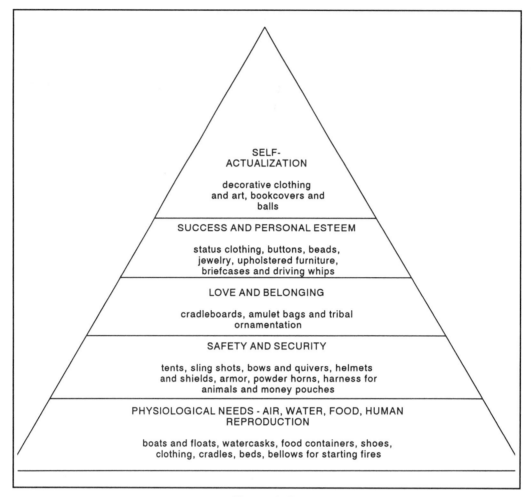

Figure 8-1.
Maslow's Hierarchy of Human Needs.

daily. In the past, leather was often used to make adaptive devices such as slings and splints for clients. Commercial products have made this, for the most part, unnecessary. However, a therapist's familiarity with leathercraft provides the knowledge to change or adapt commercial products when necessary.

ASSESSMENTS

Leatherwork is part of the following formal occupational therapy assessments:
- The Allen Cognitive Level Test, which uses a leather lacing task to determine into which of six cognitive levels a client fits. Each level is further divided into discrete functional levels (Allen, Earhart, Blue, 1992).
- The Allen Diagnostic Module, which uses an Indian key fob as one of

24 tasks used to discriminate a client's cognitive level in the 4 to 5 range (Earhart, Allen, Blue, 1993).

- The Diagnostic Test Battery, in which a client chooses a background pattern to engrave or tool on leather. Findings from this part of the assessment have to do with tactile awareness and processing, coordination, praxis, self-concept, and effect (Androes, Dreyfus, Bloesch, 1965).

- The Jacobs Prevocational Skills assessment has a section called leather assembly. The client is asked to assemble a simple leather key ring following a demonstration by the therapist (Jacobs, 1991).

Additionally, leatherwork is included in checklist evaluations such as the Neuropsychiatric Institute (NPI) Interest Checklist (Matsutsuya, 1969). The Table of Evaluations and Their Craft Components (see Table 7-1) shows what other crafts may be included in each assessment.

CHOOSING LEATHER

Leather comes from fir- and wool-bearing mammals, from scaly creatures like snakes, alligators, and lizards, and from birds such as the ostrich. Most occupational therapists who use leather choose to use cowhide, as it is versatile and less expensive than other leathers. The unit by which it is sold is the square foot. The thickness of the leather is expressed by weight in ounces, for example: 2- to 3-ounce weight leather is approximately 1/16-inch thick, 7- to 8-ounce leather is approximately 1/8-inch thick. The weights are usually given in a range of two numbers because leather is variable in thickness even on the same piece. Many occupational therapists stock two weights: 4 to 5 ounces for wallets and small projects, and 8 to 9 ounces for belts, purses, and holsters. For the modern clinic, these two choices plus a variety of precut, prepunched kits provide the optimal selection.

Kits offer an option that is hard to ignore. They certainly save the therapist's time, and consequently money, as well as sometimes their sanity when working in a busy clinic. If a therapist decides to buy and prepare all her own projects or assist clients to do so, she may stock the weights of leather described above as well as lining leather, which is a different weight and texture,in addition to a large range of laces, snaps, and fasteners. A clinic treating different levels of clients will stock both cowhide for the high-functioning client who can benefit from the challenge of starting from scratch, as well as a precut pre-punched kit that can sometimes have a pre-embossed design for the more disabled client who can successfully complete this type of kit. Availability of project kits as well as skins of tooling leather allows the therapist to grade projects appropriately for clients' functional level.

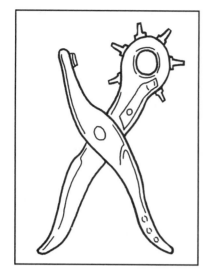

Figure 8-2.
Rotary punch.

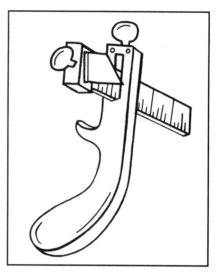

Figure 8-3.
Strap cutter.

Tools

There is such a variety of leather tools available that it is sometimes difficult to decide which ones to acquire. Nice leatherwork can be achieved with minimal tools:

- A rotary punch with replaceable cutting tubes (Figure 8-2)
- A 1 3/4 x 3 1/4-inch rawhide mallet
- A 3/4-inch oblong slotting punch
- A strap cutter (Figure 8-3)
- A snap setter
- An awl (Figure 8-4)
- Leather shears
- A utility knife
- A skife (Figure 8-5)
- A ruler
- A thonging chisel (Figure 8-6)
- Round drive punches
- An edge creaser
- A swivel knife (Figure 8-7)
- A sponge and water dish
- A tracing modeler
- Lacing needles

The six basic leathercraft stamps are:
1. The veiner (Figure 8-8)
2. The seeder (Figure 8-9)
3. The camouflage (Figure 8-10)

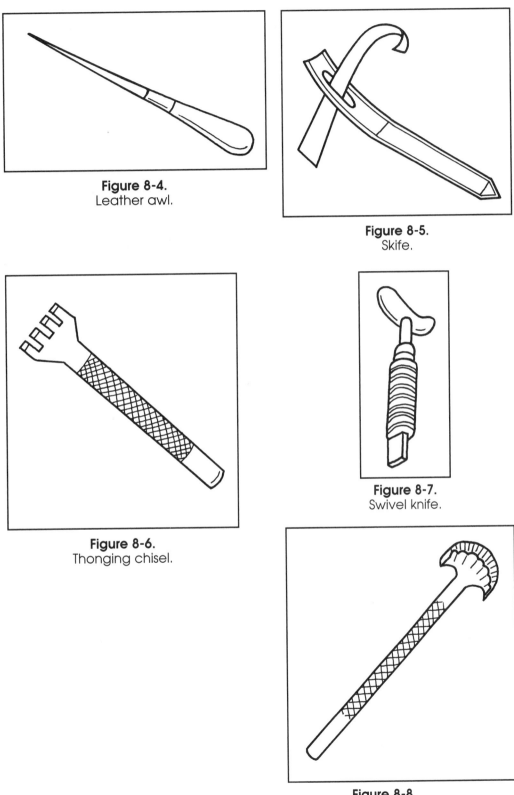

Figure 8-4.
Leather awl.

Figure 8-5.
Skife.

Figure 8-6.
Thonging chisel.

Figure 8-7.
Swivel knife.

Figure 8-8.
Veiner.

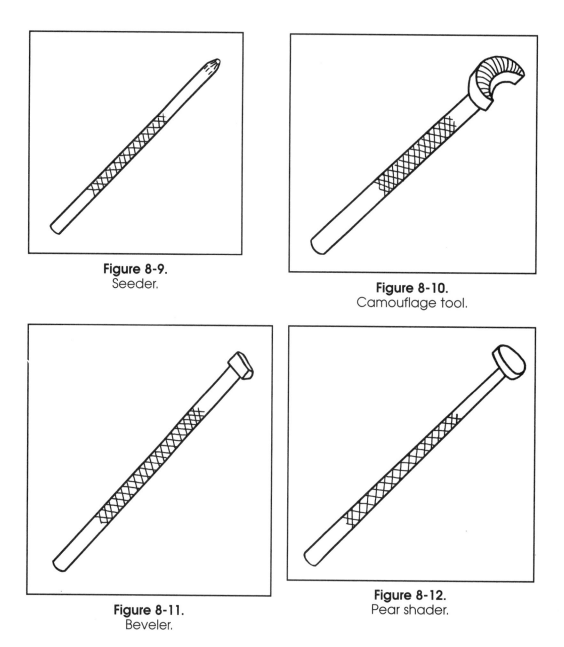

Figure 8-9.
Seeder.

Figure 8-10.
Camouflage tool.

Figure 8-11.
Beveler.

Figure 8-12.
Pear shader.

4. The beveler (Figure 8-11)
5. The pear shader (Figure 8-12)
6. The background tool (Figure 8-13)

The last three items come in a variety of textures, such as smooth, lined, or criss-crossed. The six stamping tools can achieve many interesting and attractive effects. Other decorative techniques involve the use of plastic design templates that offer an inexpensive source for attractive designs that are quick, easy, and reusable. Alphabet stamps are good for personalizing designs to emphasize a client's identity. From this basic col-

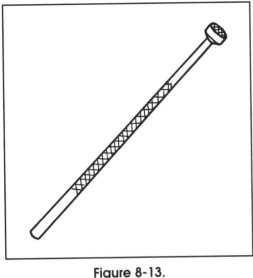

Figure 8-13.
Background tool.

lection, a therapist can gradually expand the choices as new tools and materials become available. Certain symbols, such as the peace sign in the 1960s or the unicorn in the 1980s, should be avoided, as they may become a fad.

Process

1. Select the design. If it is copied from a book rather than from a template, trace it with a pencil.
2. Cut the leather to the proper size.
3. Moisten the leather on the flesh (rough) side first and then on the grain (smooth) side with a damp (not wet) sponge. The grain side of the leather is observed until it returns to its original color. This will take a minute or less.
4. Place the traced design on the leather pencil side up so that the pencil lead does not stain the leather.
5. With the pointed end of the tracing modeler, lightly press the design into the leather.
6. Allow the leather to dry somewhat, as wet leather tends to catch on the swivel knife and cause small tears and unevenness in the line. When using the swivel knife, the leather should be just slightly damp so the knife can glide more smoothly.
7. Using a swivel knife requires practice. While the leather is drying, the client has the opportunity to practice leather carving with a swivel knife on a piece of scrap leather.
8. After all lines are carved, the leather is again moistened with a damp sponge in preparation for tooling the design.
9. Stamping tools are held upright and struck on the flat top with a rawhide mallet. The beveler (see Figure 8-11) is usually used first. The pointed end or toe of the beveling surface is placed in the cut made by the swivel knife facing toward the center of the design. Wrist and arm movements are used, rather than fingers, to manipulate the mallet in tapping the beveler as it moves along the carved line.
10. Use of the camouflage tool's half-moon shape (see Figure 8-10) is usually the next step in a tooled design.
11. Next, use the pear shader (see Figure 8-12) to create contours and shading.
12. The veiner is commonly used in nature designs, as its name comes from its similarity to leaf veins (see Figure 8-8).

13. The seeder is a small round design (see Figure 8-9) used for putting centers in flowers or similar motifs.
14. Use the background tool (see Figure 8-13) to impress the area around the design, thus causing it to stand out more dramatically. Each of these tools is held upright and tapped with the rawhide mallet. Clients may be tempted to use a steel-headed hammer. This should be avoided as it damages the chrome finish on the leatherworking tools. The steel-headed hammer can also cause the tool to puncture the leather.

These same stamping tools can be used by the clients to invent their own designs. They should practice this on a piece of scrap leather before attempting their own design on their project. A wide variety of stamping tools are available. Some are just shapes. Many are realistic pictures of objects and animals. They usually do not require the skill and concentration of leather tooling. This allows a lower functioning client an opportunity to successfully choose and create pleasing designs.

COLORING LEATHER

The natural color of leather is one of its attractions. Nonetheless, clients frequently desire to add color to their designs. There are a number of coloring agents, dyes, and acrylic paints. Clients should be encouraged to practice on scrap leather before attempting it on their project. This can be used as a lesson in life: to sample something before making a commitment that is irreversible. Each coloring agent has its own way of covering an area. It is important for the therapist and client to read the label. Color can be applied by a brush, a felt or wool dauber, or a fine-grained sponge. Moisture-resistant finishes are numerous: lacquers, waxes, and vegetable stains with an antique appearance. Oil treatment with neat's-foot or mink oil will waterproof leather, slightly darkening it. All finishes should be applied before pieces are assembled or laced.

LACING

For the occupational therapist, lacing is a particularly important part of leatherwork because its performance may indicate tactile awareness, strength, motor control, praxis, dexterity, visual awareness and perception, sequencing, and frustration tolerance. As mentioned previously, the commonly used Allen Cognitive Levels Test relies heavily on the client's lacing performance. Because of the variety of stitches—running stitch (Figure 8-14), whip stitch (Figure 8-15), single cordovan lacing (Figure 8-16), and double cordovan lacing (Figure 8-17)—it is easy to grade stitching either up to more complex or down to simple for a client who has regressed.

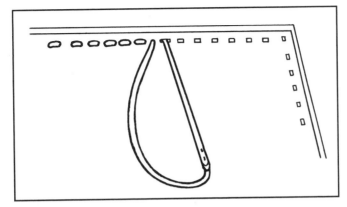

Figure 8-14.
Running stitch.

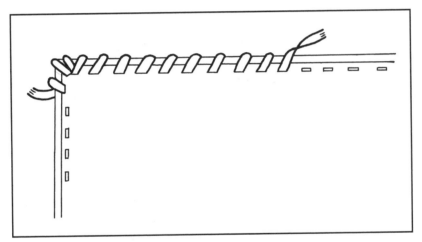

Figure 8-15.
Whip stitch.

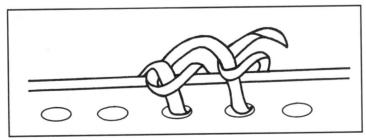

Figure 8-16.
Single cordovan lacing.

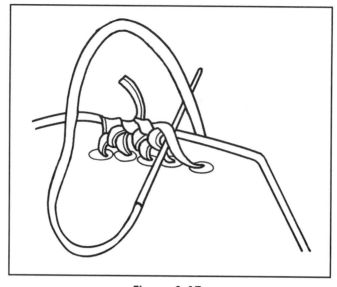

Figure 8-17.
Double cordovan lacing.

Process

1. Glue the pieces together with a thin layer of rubber cement applied to the edges of the surfaces to be joined. Avoid getting cement on anything but those surfaces.
2. Mark the line 1/8 to 1/4 of an inch from the edge with a ruler and the pointed end of the tracing modeler to indicate where lacing holes will be.
3. Use scrap wood under the leather and place the thonging chisel (see Figure 8-6) 1/4 to 1/8 of an inch from the corner on the line.
4. Hit the chisel on the head with a rawhide mallet until the cutting chisels go through to the wood and can be seen on the other side. Care must be taken to hit the chisel hard enough to make the lacing slots without cutting the leather in between. The chisel must be held perpendicular to the leather.
5. Continue making these slots wherever lacing will be used.
6. Two types of needles are commonly used: the two-prong needle (Figure 8-18) and the life-eye (Figure 8-19), which does not have a traditional eye. The pointed leather lace is screwed into the threaded open end of the life-eye needle. Less commonly used are regular large-eye needles with waxed linen or nylon thread. The type of stitching chosen will determine the difficulty of the next step. The lacing pony (Figure 8-20) is a tool for stabilizing a project for one-handed lacing. The pony is placed between the client's legs with the leather held in the clamp at a comfortable working level.

The specific instructions for each individual stitch are beyond the

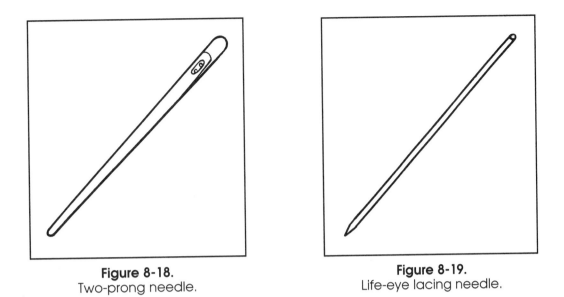

Figure 8-18.
Two-prong needle.

Figure 8-19.
Life-eye lacing needle.

scope of this book. They can be found in several of the texts listed as references at the end of this chapter. Link-belt kits are frequently used. Kits usually include precut pieces, a buckle, and the preset snap-together buckle connector and keeper, which is the slot through which the end of the belt slips after going through the buckle.

MAIN THERAPEUTIC APPLICATIONS

Physically Disabled

For the treatment of the physically disabled, leathercraft is gradable from simple to complex. It is not messy compared to wood or clay; it can be carried easily by a therapist for use with bed patients. The project will not be damaged if the client's endurance limit is reached and the project stopped. It can be started again at almost any point. For clients in infectious disease isolation, leathercraft is an option since most leather tools can be disinfected. (Steel rotary punches may rust if not completely dried after immersion in liquid.) The leather, however, is difficult to sterilize. Chemicals in disinfectants may affect tanned leather color and suppleness. Wet leather will shrink like wet shoes dried on a heat vent. Simple projects that require few tools such as link belts or prestamped kits ready to be laced are an easy alternative for isolated clients.

For physically disabled clients who need upper extremity strengthening and increased endurance, leatherwork offers many opportunities. Cutting leather uses finger and thumb flexors and extensors, forearm supinators, and shoulder extensors. Using the swivel knife requires static pinch, finger and thumb adduction and opposition, and wrist, ulnar, and radial deviation. Tooling and stamping use finger and thumb flexion,

opposition and pinch, and wrist flexion and extension. Gripping a rotary
punch requires finger and thumb flexion. Lacing involves most muscle
groups—finger and thumb flexion,
opposition, wrist flexion and extension, pronation and supination, elbow
flexion and extension, shoulder flexion and extension, abduction, and
external rotation. Leatherwork can be
a good method of achieving these
strengthening goals while using purposeful activity to produce a pleasing
product. Strengthening is achieved by
gradually increasing the amount of
force needed to perform the action.
Slings, mobile arm supports, and the
lacing pony can assist weakened
joints and muscles.

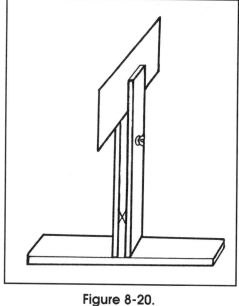

Figure 8-20.
Lacing pony.

The sight-impaired client can use
leathercraft as a way of increasing
tactile awareness, the same tactile awareness required in using Braille
reading and writing. As the client works on the design, the impressions
and contours can be felt with the fingers. The skills learned in working
with leathercraft can be transferred to other activities such as dialing a
telephone and identifying textures in putting clothes on right side out.

Mental Health

In the treatment of mental health clients, leather is commonly used.
Easy projects such as link-belt kits or simple lacing can easily be completed by low-functioning clients. Advancement to more complex projects
demonstrates in a very concrete way that a client's functioning is improving. Leathercraft can be used to address such common problems in mental health as attention span, memory, visual awareness and processing,
fine coordination and dexterity, self-concept, problem solving, and the
need to express unconscious feelings in a safe and structured context.
Natural products made of leather are valued for their scarcity, as our
society has come to rely increasingly on synthetics. Consequently, completion of a leather item can enhance self-esteem and self-concept, which
is a problem for almost all psychiatric clients. Traditionally, leatherwork
has been a male-oriented craft. It continues to be useful in that way,
although many female clients enjoy it too.

Benefits for the mentally retarded come in the areas of fine coordination, dexterity, and concentration in both stamping and lacing. Lacing
and stamping include both fine and gross motor control. The necessity to
pay attention to where one puts the needle and where one places the

leather stamp requires concentration. Increasing concentration occurs by gradually increasing the amount of time spent on the task.

Pediatrics

Leatherwork is seldom used by younger, acute care, physically disabled clients. By the time children are well enough to do leatherwork, they are usually discharged from the hospital. Older children and teenagers are more likely to use leather. Kits offer satisfactory projects for pediatrics, as leathercraft is not used often enough to spend the time it takes to buy and cut the leather. Some therapists report that they seldom use leathercraft because children show little interest in it. However, it may be an appropriate assignment for angry children as they can sublimate anger through hammering. Leather craft should be avoided for any child who is hypersensitive to sound or touch. It can be used to evaluate coordination and attention span in children.

Geriatrics

Strength is an important consideration for leatherwork, as the elderly may have diminished vigor. Because many of the tools could cause cuts and bruises, the therapist must be observant of the clients' coordination, visual awareness, and visual processing. Cuts and bruises in some older people are difficult to heal. Many older people also have painful osteoarthritis. Gripping tools either in a pinch or grasp may aggravate the arthritis. Leather is considered by some to be a male-identified craft, and nine out of 10 elders are females, which may be why leathercraft is less often used than needlework, cooking, or other "female" crafts for elderly women clients.

CASE STUDY

Rafael is a 23-year-old Mexican-American male who grew up in east Los Angeles. He had been brought to the county's alcohol and drug treatment unit. The police had picked him up outside a bar where he had been fighting. The bartender had difficulty putting him out. He and another customer had begun to argue about a debt Rafael owed. After Rafael had tried to pick up the barstool to hit the other customer, the bartender intervened and maneuvered him outside, locked the door, and called the police. When they arrived, Rafael was sitting up against the wall snoring. The police had taken him to a detoxification unit. After 36 hours, they sent him to the alcohol and drug rehabilitation unit.

During the screening interview, the occupational therapist learned about Rafael's background. His mother had been born in the United States when her mother and father were migrant workers in the fruit orchards of California. His father had illegally come across the Mexican border to find work. He was successful in that endeavor and met Rafael's mother in a Catholic church service center. Rafael was the youngest of their eight children. He had dropped out of high school when he was in 10th grade "because it was boring." Since that time he had worked at a variety of unskilled day labor jobs. As long as he could remember, alcohol and "machismo" had been associated with each other in Rafael's mind. While he had been arrested for drunkenness before, this was the first time he had ever undergone treatment. He was engaged to marry a family friend from his neighborhood last year. The engagement was called off after Rafael broke her jaw when he hit her during a drunken rage. Following this incident, his family asked him to leave their home, as he was an embarrassment to them. They feared his unpredictable behavior.

The occupational therapy clinic in the rehabilitation center used an eclectic theory approach, which meant that the therapist chose whichever of approximately seven assessments she thought fit the client with whom she was working. Since her screening interview had shown problems with leisure exploration, problem solving, self control, and time management, she selected evaluations she thought would analyze these components in more depth. The evaluations she chose to use with Rafael were the NPI Interest Checklist, the Activities Configuration, and the Allen Cognitive Levels Test. On the NPI Interest Checklist, he indicated a strong interest in leatherwork. On the Activities Configuration, in which he filled out a week's schedule of his pre-rehabilitation activities and marked how independent he felt about the each thing he did, he showed a very low feeling of autonomy even about the time he spent drinking.

When the therapist discussed his test with him, he reported that from an early age he had been passive in groups and allowed others to make decisions for him. He was found to be functioning at a level of 5.4 on the Allen Cognitive Levels Test. His peripheral neuropathy apparently caused some difficulty with strength and dexterity in manipulating the needle and lace. After the lacing test, he told the therapist he had always wanted to work with leather since he had seen an uncle in Mexico doing leather tooling once during a family visit.

The therapist sat down with Rafael to devise a treatment plan. Rafael told the therapist he would like to learn something that would help him get a job. After discussing the role of occupational therapy in his treatment program, they set the following goals:

- To develop a daily activity plan and schedule and carry it out during the 28-day treatment program
- To attend the daily occupational therapy goal-setting group to make and discuss achievement of daily goals
- To increase the strength and dexterity of his upper extremities

During the first week, Rafael was able to complete a leather belt with a western buckle for himself. He was pleased with the outcome and wanted to do something more complicated. For his second project, he decided to make a shoulder bag for his mother, who had come to visit him in the rehabilitation center. During this same time, he began a weight-lifting program with the recreation therapist. His strength and endurance began to show real improvement. During his last week, he decided to try to make something for his father as a peace offering. His mother told him that his father was still angry with him because of his treatment of his former fiancée. After a discussion with the therapist, he decided to design and make a tool holster for his father, who worked in construction. They used the occupational therapy wrench, pliers, and hammer to draw a pattern on newsprint paper. He drew his own decorative western design for the holster. It was made to fit on his father's belt, as he did not know his father's waist size. On the day before he was discharged, it appeared as if he would not be able to finish, so the therapist got permission from the nursing staff to allow Rafael to work on the lacing that night. He came to craft group proudly displaying the finished tool holster. During the last session, they talked as a group about what they had done during these sessions. Rafael talked hopefully about a reconciliation with his father.

DISCUSSION QUESTIONS

1. What questions might you ask Rafael at the time of his discharge to help him assess whether he had achieved his goals?
2. Can you name any other cultural group for whom leather is especially meaningful? What kinds of designs might they use?
3. If a client chose to make a 10 x 7-inch decorative book cover, what are some assumptions we might make about him or her?
4. What leather project samples do you think might be the most important to have available in the occupational therapy clinic?
5. What kinds of clients might be more likely to choose to make a project like the samples you named?

REFERENCES

Allen, C. K., Earhart, C. A., & Blue, T. (1992). *Occupational therapy treatment goals for the physically and cognitively disabled.* Rockville, MD: American Occupational Therapy Association.

Androes, L., Dreyfus, E. A., & Bloesch, M. (1965). Diagnostic test battery for occupational therapy. *Am J Occup Ther, 19*(2), 53-59.

Earhart, C. A., Allen, C. K., & Blue, T. (1993). *Allen diagnostic module.* Colchester, CT: S & S Worldwide.

Jacobs, K. (1991). *Occupational therapy: Work-related programs and assessment* (2nd ed.). Boston: Little, Brown & Company.

Matsutsuya, J. S. (1969). The interest checklist. *Am J Occup Ther, 23*(4), 323-328.

Reader's Digest. (1979). *Crafts and hobbies.* Pleasantville, NY: The Reader's Digest Association Inc.

Stohlman, A., Patten, A. D., & Wilson, J. A. (1969). *Leatherwork manual.* Fort Worth, TX: Tandy Leather Company.

NEEDLEWORK

INTRODUCTION

Needlework could include everything from sewing tanned animal hides together, to sail-making for boats, to creating fine altar clothes for churches or intricate tapestries for castle or museum walls.

In 18th and 19th century America, needlecraft was often the measure of a woman's worth. Sewing clothing for the family as well as quilting and mending were her constant occupations (Banks, 1979).

Needlework, like woodcraft, includes such a vast number of activities that limits must be defined specifically for the purposes of occupational therapy. Four needlework categories are described here.

TYPES OF NEEDLEWORK

Simple Sewing

Simple sewing includes making clothing and home furnishings. Stitches in simple sewing start with the running stitch or basting stitch, to the more difficult smocking, ruffling, and buttonhole stitches (Carroll, 1947).

Quilting is a particularly American craft for home decoration. Many stitches in quilting qualify as simple sewing though the designs and color combinations may be complex (*Reader's Digest*, 1979).

Embroidery

Embroidery is a way of making a picture or design on cloth using a needle and thread. It can be either simple or complex. There are more than 80 different embroidery stitches from which one can choose in planning a design. Different yarn or floss is used; for example, in crewel embroidery, loosely twisted yarn (usually wool) is stitched on heavier fabric (Carroll, 1947).

Knitting and Crocheting

Knitting and crocheting are both methods of using interlocking loops to make garments of clothing or articles for home use. Knitting uses two needles and is usually made in rows. Crocheting requires only one hook-like needle and stitching may be created in a round shape, squares, or in rows.

Needlepoint

Needlepoint is a variation of cross-stitch embroidery. It is done on a canvas back. Many of the world's fine tapestries are this kind of stitchery. Today's counted cross-stitch is a modern version of traditional needlepoint in which the design is worked by counting threads and coloring in the design with stitchery.

FREQUENCY OF USE

About one fifth of occupational therapy clinicians use needlework weekly. Many others occasionally use needlework in treatment. It can be considered a major tool for occupational therapists both as an activity for clients and as a method of producing adaptive equipment.

ASSESSMENTS

Needlework is included in assessment of activities of daily living and self-care more often than in assessments of thinking or creativity. Three such self-care evaluations are the Milwaukee Evaluations of Daily Living Skills (MEDLS) (Leonardelli, 1988), the Homemaking Evaluation in Occupational Therapy for Physical Dysfunction (Trombly, 1983), and the Activities of Daily Living Evaluation (Pedretti, Zoltan, 1990). The Neuropsychiatric Institute (NPI) Interest Checklist (Matsutsuya, 1969), and Activity Index (Gregory, 1983; Nystrom, 1974) also include this craft. Newer assessments for the physically disabled do not include a sewing task (Asher, 1996).

The MEDLS is an assessment of daily living skills for the chronically mentally ill. It has 20 subtest categories. In the MEDLS, under the category *Maintenance of Clothing*, clients are given a needle, thread, scissors, and a shirt with a button missing and are told to sew on the button. They are scored on whether they are able to complete all or part of the task in each subtest category (Leonardelli, 1988).

The Homemaking Evaluation (Trombly, 1983), designed to be used in rehabilitation settings, includes sewing as one of seven major areas. The evaluation is a checklist to be completed by the therapist at the beginning of rehabilitation treatment and again at discharge. It is administered over several sessions.

The Activities of Daily Living Evaluation contains a section on hand activities that include basting and sewing on a button. This evaluation was adapted from one used at the Hartford Easter Seal Center (Pedretti, Zoltan, 1990).

The NPI Interest Checklist is filled out by the client. It asks the client to rate his or her interest as casual, strong, or none in 80 activities. Sewing, needlework, mending, and knitting are on the list. Two other activities—decorating and making clothes—may include needlework (Matsutsuya, 1969).

The Activity Index for people over age 65 is a questionnaire with 61 questions about participation and the importance of 25 different leisure activities/occupations. The activities/occupations are rated for frequency of participation, level of interest and enjoyment, self-reported skill level, and whether the client does it on his or her own volition or whether he or she feels required to do it (Gregory, 1983; Nystrom, 1974). Informal needlework evaluations can identify functional levels of eye-hand coordination, fine motor coordination, dexterity, sequencing, and praxis.

Supplies

One of the simplest stitches used in kits is cross-stitch. It has a long history with people who tried to improve their eye-hand and fine motor skills. Many 18th century girlhood samplers used mostly cross-stitch (Banks, 1979; Creekmore, 1968). While a high-functioning client may be able to concentrate to count the stitches for the popular counted cross-stitch patterns, many clients will find it too difficult. The stamped cross-stitch kit or precut plastic canvas that has preprinted color codes offers a good alternative. Additional tools needed in needlework are both left- and right-handed scissors; thimbles; different sizes of embroidery hoops, including a three-way hoop that can stand on a table, be held between legs, or clamped to a table and used by one-handed clients (Figure 9-1); and an assortment of embroidery and crewel needles.

Process

1. Place the bottom section of the hoop under the part of the stamped design where you want to start.
2. Press the top of the hoop over the cloth and the inner hoop. This stretches the fabric so it is easy to see the design.

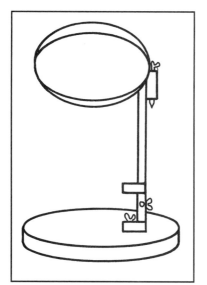

Figure 9-1.
Three-way
embroidery hoop.

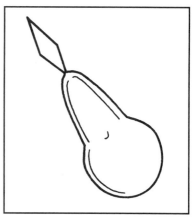

Figure 9-2.
Needle threader.

3. Cut off a 14-inch piece of cotton embroidery floss (made up of six strands of thread).
4. Separate the six strands in two so there are two strands with three threads in each
5. Thread the needle. Embroidery needles have larger eyes so all strands can fit through. It may be necessary to use a needle threader, which is an important aid for most clinics (Figure 9-2). Pull the thread one third of the way through.
6. Knot the longest side on the end. Expert embroiderers do not knot their threads, but for most clients it is necessary to knot the thread to keep it from pulling through.
7. From the back of the cloth, push the needle up through the end of one cross and down on the other end: then up on the other line of the same cross and down (Figure 9-3).
8. Continue this process on each cross.
9. When the thread gets short (approximately 4 inches) make a knot by going over and under floss strands on the back several times.
10. Cut off the excess thread, leaving 1/4 to 1/2 inch after the knot.
11. Change floss colors as indicated on the schematic directions included in the kit.
12. Move the hoop when the thread gets too close to the edge to work comfortably.
13. When the stitching is finished, remove the hoop.
14. Iron the picture flat. It is then ready to frame, to be sewn to a pillow cover, or otherwise finished.

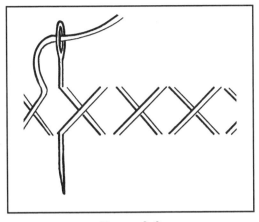

Figure 9-3.
Cross-stitch with an embroidery needle.

To add more complexity, clients can draw their own design and transfer it to embroidery cloth or canvas. Another way to vary a design is to use applique. A figure cut from one kind of fabric is sewn to another piece of cloth. A variety of stitches may be used to stitch the figure down. It can be stitched down using a buttonhole stitch on the sewing machine or by hand (Creekmore, 1968).

MAIN THERAPEUTIC APPLICATIONS

Physical Dysfunction

Because needlework is most often identified with women, its use is slightly limited. While a few men will attempt it; only those with a strong sense of self are willing to risk doing a traditionally female craft (Department of the Army, 1971). Needlework is the kind of craft that can be done easily by bed patients. Small projects require little expenditure of energy and can be done by very weak clients. It can be stopped whenever the client is fatigued and started when the client is refreshed. Because the materials are inexpensive, they can be left in the rooms of clients in infectious isolation. Scissors can be easily sterilized with disinfectants if necessary. The therapist needs to make sure the scissors are completely dry after sterilizing so they do not rust.

Most of the joint and muscle movements in needlecraft are in the fingers and hands. However, needlework involves some shoulder internal and external rotation, elbow flexion and extension, forearm pronation and supination, wrist flexion and extension, and radial and ulnar deviation. Many severely disabled arthritics still enjoy needlework, as it does not require strength and consequently does not hurt their joints. The client experiences less pain when concentrating on a craft such as needlework (Council on Physical Medicine of the American Medical Association, 1947).

If an arthritic client uses a joint continuously in position, it is possible for the stress to further damage an inflamed joint. Precautions need to be taken to avoid this. This craft is not good for the visually impaired, as they cannot see patterns to stitch.

Mental Health

Embroidery can be very structured, as in cross-stitch, or it can be a challenging, creative experience. For depressed, low-functioning clients, needlework can be used in the acute stage of the illness, as it requires little exertion. Most depressed clients complain of fatigue, but needlework is seldom a fatiguing activity. Historically, people have used it for relaxation, such as in quilting. For hostile clients, the cutting and piercing parts of the needlework process may help them turn their hostility to constructive use. The striving for repetition and preoccupation with detail that afflicts the obsessive compulsive client can be easily satisfied through needlecraft. Stitchery can make constructive use of these otherwise negative behaviors. The mentally retarded can enjoy and benefit from the repetitive possibilities of needlework. They can learn one step and repeat it many times.

Pediatrics

Young children ages 5 to 6 years may not have received the message that this is a female craft. It is valuable for both sexes, as it involves many perceptual and fine motor skills that children need to develop, such as eye-hand coordination. Sewing cards or cardboard with perforated holes along the outline of the picture are often used for beginning sewers. While it can be repetitious, it need not be. Perhaps the best way to present it to children is that stitchery is another way of drawing or picture making. They can be encouraged to draw an outline on cloth and then stitch on that line. Burlaps or other coarse cloths are appropriate for children's stitchery. Large plastic needles are good to use on burlap. Other less coarse cloth requires metal needles that should be used cautiously, as they are usually sharp. If a therapist is going to do such a project with a group of children, it may be best to cut the yarn and thread all the needles before the children arrive, as they are seldom able to sit and wait for their turn for help from the therapist in threading their needle (Gaitskell, Hurwitz, 1975). Projects appropriate for children of different ages as well as adolescents include wall hangings, hand puppets, placemats, or simple doll clothes. Children enjoy embellishing their creations with beads, buttons, sequins, and iron-on patches.

Geriatrics

Many elderly females have sewn and mended for themselves and their families throughout their lives. While women will often do a traditional male craft, few men will participate in female-identified crafts such as needlework. Because women have habitually stitched from necessity and for recreation, as in quilting, it is usually easy to get them to participate. They may also have a preferred type of needlecraft that they have done in the past. If so, this is probably the best medium for them to work in (Gould, Gould, 1971). If vision is a problem, as it often is for the elderly, using bright colors on white will be helpful. The contrast makes it easier for them to see. A clamp-on magnifying glass may be attached to the edge of the table if necessary. People with circulation problems, common in diabetes, need to be careful not to stick themselves with the needles as they may develop infections. Sometimes demented elderly use scissors to damage something, such as cutting their own clothes or bed linens. Precautions should be taken to prevent this.

CASE STUDY

Alice was 49 years old when she discovered a lump in her right breast. She had gotten out of the habit of breast self-examination after she went to work. Consequently, her breast cancer was quite advanced when the biopsy was done and the cancer was diagnosed. Cancer was found in her axial lymph nodes. Because Alice had not agreed to a radical mastectomy before the biopsy, she had to be rehospitalized for this major surgery. Her local surgeon referred her to a cancer specialty hospital in a nearby city.

The occupational therapist there was an important member of the treatment team. She paid a visit to Alice for a screening interview the day before Alice was to undergo the radical mastectomy. This was considered an important part of the preventive medicine emphasized in the specialty hospital. The therapist hoped to prevent postsurgical complications. She learned that Alice had four daughters and worked as a bookkeeper before she was married. After the girls were in school, she did the bookkeeping for her husband's farm feed and seed store. When she was 46, her husband divorced her and married a local school teacher. Alice had been devastated by this unexpected turn of events. For a year, she kept working in the business of her ex-husband because she was afraid she was not skilled enough to do the complex computer bookkeeping required in most businesses. A friend persuaded her to take a computer class at the local junior college. Her computer teacher helped her find a job in the client accounts department of the local hospital. Several months later she discovered the lump in her breast. Her daughters rallied to her support. Three of them lived within 50 miles.

The occupational therapist queried Alice about her hobbies and learned that she had sewn many of her girls' clothes as they grew up. Recently, she had been making doll clothes for her 6-year-old granddaughter. They agreed that doll clothes might be a good activity for her to continue to work on during the 5 to 10 days she was expected to be in the hospital. The occupational therapy department used two main theories to guide treatment: Lifestyle/Adaptive Performance and the Rehabilitation Model. The occupational therapist and Alice made the following goals:

- To prevent right shoulder contracture
- To prevent right upper extremity edema
- To prevent depression

The occupational therapist visited Alice soon after she returned to her hospital room from the recovery room. The next day, after checking her range of motion, she started Alice on some mild shoulder exercises and helped her cut out the pieces for a doll dress. Alice was medicated for pain. The occupational therapist instructed Alice about steps to take to prevent edema and infection in her right arm. Needle punctures needed to be avoided, as they could cause infection. Since her lymphatic system in that arm had been interrupted, she was much more vulnerable to wound infection, which could be quite serious for her. Alice's surgical incision was healing well. She worked much of the time on the doll wardrobe for her granddaughter. She immediately became involved in a mastectomy patients' support group. At the time of discharge, she had increased her shoulder flexion 15° since the day after surgery. From time to time, when Alice returned to the cancer specialty hospital for her chemotherapy and radiation treatments, she visited her occupational therapist. She appeared to have adapted well to her condition. Sewing had become a social enabler for her, as she was now making doll clothes to be sold in a church bazaar.

DISCUSSION QUESTIONS

1. What craft might the occupational therapist have suggested that would have involved shoulder flexion so that Alice could have used an activity rather than an exercise to achieve this movement?
2. Which needlecraft would be the least likely to cause a needle puncture wound?
3. If Alice had developed a staphylococcus infection in her surgical incision and was put into isolation so other clients could not contract the infection from her, as is sometimes the case, what would you do so that she could continue to participate in this activity, which was so good for her?

REFERENCES

Asher, I. E. (1996). *Occupational therapy assessment tools: An annotated index* (2nd ed.). Bethesda, MD: American Occupational Therapy Association.

Banks, M. (1979). *Anonymous was a woman.* New York: St. Martinis Press.

Carroll, A. (1947). *The good house keeping needlecraft encyclopedia.* New York: Rinehart & Company.

Council on Physical Medicine of the American Medical Association. (1947). *Manual of occupational therapy.* Chicago: American Medical Association.

Creekmore, B. B. (1968). *Traditional American crafts.* New York: Hearthside Press.

Department of the Army. (1971). *Craft techniques in occupational therapy* Washington, DC: U.S. Government Printing Office.

Gaitskell, C. D., & Hurwitz, A. (1975). *Children and their art* (3rd ed.). New York: Harcourt, Brace, Jovanovitch.

Gould, E., & Gould, L. (1971). *Crafts for the elderly.* Springfield, IL: Charles C.Thomas Publisher.

Gregory, M. D. (1983). Occupational behavior and life satisfaction among retirees. *Am J Occup Ther, 37*(8), 548-553.

Leonardelli, C. A. (1988). *The Milwaukee evaluation of daily living skills: Evaluation in long-term psychiatric care.* Thorofare, NJ: SLACK Incorporated.

Matsutsuya, J. S. (1969). The interest checklist. *Am J Occup Ther, 24*(4).

Nystrom, E. P. (1974). Activity patterns and leisure concepts among the elderly. *Am J Occup Ther, 28*(4): 337-345.

Pedretti, L. S., & Zoltan, B. (1990). *Occupational therapy: Practice skills for physical dysfunction.* St. Louis: Mosby.

Reader's Digest. (1979). *Crafts and hobbies.* Pleasantville, NY: The Reader's Digest Association Inc.

Trombly, C. A. (1983). *Occupational therapy for physical dysfunction* (2nd ed.). Baltimore: Waverly Press.

COPPER TOOLING AND METAL CRAFT

INTRODUCTION

While metal and its uses were discovered by humans thousands of years after wood, ceramics, and leather, it was such an important development that we have named an era after it—the Iron Age, as compared with the Stone Age or Computer Age. Metalworking has existed at least 12,000 years. Copper, along with gold, probably was discovered first. Copper is an element that is very malleable. It was hammered into utilitarian and decorative objects. The copper tooling we do today has a long history of use (*Reader's Digest*, 1979). Other metals such as gold, silver, bronze, iron, pewter, and aluminum have been crafted, but in modern occupational therapy clinics, copper and tin are most likely to be used. Tin is also an elemental metal. The occupational therapists' use of these two metals will be emphasized in this chapter.

FREQUENCY OF USE

In studies of crafts used by occupational therapists, there were two categories that involved metal craft: metal hammering and copper tooling. Many clinics use metal craft (Arris, Cordero, Christiaansen, 1986; Titus, 1997). This makes it an important skill for new therapists to have.

ASSESSMENTS

No formal assessments were found to include metal work. Because metal work is new to most clients, they would have to learn every step before it could be performed. Consequently, this probably requires more time than many therapists have for the evaluation process and could narrow the range of skills that could be evaluated. Danger may also be considered as a factor for excluding metal work in task evaluation batteries. Clients could very easily cut themselves on the sharp metal edges.

TYPES OF METAL CRAFTS

Tooling is a method of making a design on a sheet of metal foil. Metal foil comes in copper, aluminum, silver, and gold-colored aluminum. The thickness of the metal foil or sheet is expressed in the term *gauge*. Most tooling is done on 30- to 40-gauge metal. The thicker the foil, the lower the number. Copper is most commonly used probably because of its malleability and stretchability.

Embossing is a method of working the metal from the back of the foil to raise the design on the front. Chasing is the same process but done from the front of the foil. When both are combined to get a picture, it is called repousse, which means worked from both sides. All three of these methods are included in the term *copper tooling* (*Reader's Digest*, 1979).

Metal can also be soldered, riveted, cut, bent, etched, cast, or enameled. Because of the infrequency of use of most of these techniques in occupational therapy, they will not be further explained here.

Tooling

SUPPLIES
- 36-gauge sheet copper
- Tracing paper and pencil
- Plastic picture templates
- Plasticine clay
- Steel wool
- Liver of sulfur
- Water
- Lacquer
- Lacquer thinner
- Masking tape
- Newspapers

TOOLS
- A modeling tool (leather tracing modeler can be used)
- Sharpened hardwood dowels for tracing
- Tongue depressor
- Brush for liver of sulfur
- Brush for lacquer

- Dish for liver of sulfur
- Dish for brush cleaning
- Metal shears

The process described here will be for clients using their own designs, however the process of using templates is similar, but simpler.

Process

1. Trace the design onto the tracing paper.
2. Cut the copper to the correct size.
3. Cover all the edges with masking tape to prevent cuts from sharp edges.
4. Tape the tracing paper to the metal.
5. Place this on a 1-inch thick stack of newspapers.
6. Use the sharpened wooden dowel to trace evenly over all the lines to lightly impress the design into the metal foil.
7. Remove the tracing paper.
8. Retrace the line with the blunt point of the modeling tool.
9. Turn the copper over. Next, use the spoon end of the modeling tool (or a dowel with a rounded end) and, starting in the middle, slowly and evenly press all the parts of the design that are to be raised. Starting at the edge may cause folds in the metal. Avoid working in only one area, as that copper will stretch and wrinkle. Work over the whole area.
10. Turn the copper over frequently so the raised design is facing up and flatten out the background by pressing it against the hard table top with the same tool. Alternate, working on the front and back. The important thing to remember is to work slowly and evenly over the whole area to avoid stretching one section more or making a hole in the copper.
11. When the design is raised to its completed height, fill in the reverse side of the impression with plasticine (an oil-based clay), smoothing the clay slowly and evenly to fill in the back of the raised surface.
12. Turn the copper over and with a pointed tool, gently impress in the detailed lines of the design on the front.
13. Lightly go over the front of the copper with fine steel wool to clean off any dirt or oil left from the tooling process. Be careful not to touch the copper after this, as body oil will resist the liver of sulfur (described in step 15).
14. Most liver of sulfur comes in a solution form, but if it is purchased in lump form, dissolve a pea-sized lump in one quart of water.
15. Dip the copper in this solution, or if the copper is too big to fit in the pan it can be applied with a brush. Liver of sulfur fumes can

be unpleasant, as it is the typical rotten egg smell. People with allergies or respiratory problems need to be careful to avoid these fumes.

16. After the metal is dry, buff the front of the design with fine steel wool. This will allow the black oxidation from the liver of sulfur to remain in the crevices and provide contrast for the raised design.
17. After the desired polish and contrast is achieved on the front, the piece should be covered with a thin layer of lacquer that can be applied with a brush or as a spray.
18. The lacquer brush should be cleaned with lacquer thinner followed by soap and water.

Tooling done on plastic templates is the same except it leaves out the steps of tracing on paper and onto the copper because the design is already on the plastic template. Tape the copper to either the front or back of the template, whichever side has the greatest detail. Press the copper into the grooves and depressions of the template by first going over the whole surface with a blunt tool or tongue depressor, working from the middle toward the edges. Then, gradually decrease the bluntness of the tool and begin to emphasize the details. If the design seems indistinct in any sections, turn the template over to see what details need to be emphasized. For the lower-functioning client, it may be better to tape the copper to the back of the template so the depressed design can be filled with clay before it is removed from the template. Otherwise, the process is the same (Department of the Army, 1971; Griswold, 1931). The finished tooling may be mounted on wood using copper escutcheon pins, or it can be placed in a picture frame.

Hammering

Hammering a flat metal sheet into a shape is called planishing. The process toughens the copper and gives it a texture. The tools and supplies for this process are minimal.

TOOLS AND SUPPLIES

- Concave wooden mold
- Rawhide, rubber, or wooden mallet
- 20- to 24-gauge copper disk

PROCESS

1. Center the copper disk on the mold.
2. With a few blows of the mallet, define the edge of the concave area under the disk (Figure 10-1).
3. Hit with the hammer, moving in a spiral outward from the center until the desired shape and texture are reached (*Reader's Digest*, 1979; Department of the Army, 1971).

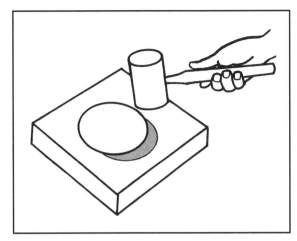

Figure 10-1.
Mallet, copper disk, and wooden mold.

An alternative method of hammering that reduces the noise made by using a wooden mold is to use a cloth sandbag. Nestle the copper or other metal disk into the sandbag, similar to the way a person sits in a beanbag chair. Use a rubber mallet to tap the disk into a concave shape. The disk may need to be repositioned in the sandbag as the work progresses.

Chasing and Piercing

Chasing means making an indention on the front of the piece without actually piercing the metal. Another kind of metalworking is nail punching or piercing of the design. Both can be done on either copper or tin sheets, on tin pie plates, or tin coasters.

TOOLS AND SUPPLIES
- A Phillips screwdriver or nail and hammer
- A piece of scrap wood
- A traced design

PROCESS
1. Affix the traced design to the top surface of the metal.
2. Place the metal on the wood.
3. Depending on the thickness of the metal and whether chasing or piercing of the design is planned, use either a sharp nail for piercing or a blunt nail or Phillips screwdriver for chasing. Position the nail or screwdriver and gently tap it.
4. Repeat until the outline of the design is complete.

Experimenting on a scrap of metal is recommended before actually starting to work on the design. Nail punching is in an old American craft used in making the panels on pie safes and other food storage cupboards.

It lets air in but keeps mice and roaches out. Nail punching kits offer opportunities to create objects that look antique. Some therapists call this technique *nail art* (Johnson, Lobdell, Nesbitt, Clare, 1996).

MAIN THERAPEUTIC APPLICATIONS

Physical Dysfunction

Often a goal in tooling is to strengthen finger and hand flexors and the three-jaw chuck grip. Adaptations for poor grip can easily be made by using built-up tools, using a larger sharpened dowel for a modeling tool or using lighter gauge metal. Because of the concentrated static contraction of finger and hand muscles, a client may need frequent rest periods. Even a client who has poor muscle strength and control in the hand can achieve nice results. It is a quiet activity that requires little space. Clients using only one hand can perform this craft. The therapist will need to tape down the design to be traced as well as the paper for the metal tracing. A template can also be taped in place for the one-handed client. Liver of sulfur, steel wool, and lacquer can also be applied in the same way. Clients will need to use gloves to protect their hands when using steel wool. Those for whom infection is a major threat, such as diabetics, need to have special precautions taken because copper tooling has so many hazards for skin cuts or punctures on the sharp metal edges or from the steel wool. Liver of sulfur is corrosive to the airways and skin, so it is best to use it in a well-ventilated space while wearing gloves. It may be necessary for the therapist to apply the liver of sulfur in a room away from clients with respiratory ailments. Copper tooling either with a template or the client's own design can be used with blind or partially sighted clients. They can feel the contours of the picture in the same way they feel the dots for reading Braille. Again, precautions need to be taken to cover all sharp edges with masking tape, as the blind person is unable to visually observe the dangers. Bed patients can do copper tooling, but it may be advisable to use the liver of sulfur and steel wool out of the bed on a bedside table.

Hammering a metal sheet into a mold involves elbow flexors and extension, as well as ulnar and radial deviation. These motions need to be chosen with care so that a weak joint is not overtaxed or inflamed by excessive motion or impact (Department of the Army, 1951; 1971; Dunton, 1945; McCann, 1978; Rich, 1960).

Mental Health

Because copper tooling on templates is a success-assured activity, many occupational therapists in psychiatric settings use it. Self-esteem is a problem for a large number of psychiatric clients, and copper tooling offers a project with a successful outcome—success is tied to self-esteem.

This craft can be graded from a simple, small template to a larger, more complex template; from a simple, traced design, to a more complex design and finally to a creative design composed by the client. Copper tooling can be used to focus on attention span, ability to stay within limits, to sequence steps, or to make decisions. If a variety of templates are available to choose from, clients who feel many choices have been denied them in the hospital find themselves in a situation where they can exert some control. A client with destructive behavior may find this rather controlled destructive/constructive craft to be a good way to sublimate harmful hostile urges. For the depressed client, the no-fail aspect of copper tooling may be the most important. Most depressed clients have some measure of decreased self-esteem. This activity usually will not let them fail again. The slow repetitive movements are the ones depressed clients are able to do despite their fatigue. The sharp edges of the copper, however, may be a temptation for self-injurious or suicidal clients. Clients who undergo electro-convulsive therapy (ECT) who may have memory problems will have little difficulty with this simple craft (Ayers, 1949).

In the case of some schizophrenics, the structure offered by tooling a template is helpful. The limits are well-defined for those schizophrenics for whom boundaries are difficult to perceive. The activity does not require much concentration or thinking, processes that are difficult for some schizophrenics. The here-and-now quality of this activity, in which the client is able to see immediate results, often helps schizophrenic clients exercise their own reality testing. Clients with organic mental disorders benefit from copper tooling for many of the same reasons as schizophrenics—it requires few cognitive processes and yet provides a good outcome for the client.

Manic clients who have expansive behaviors can have inherent controls for their hyperactivity. The obvious guidelines of a template help them provide a control for themselves. The resistiveness of the copper can provide a controlled outlet for excess energy. The clients can quickly complete the activity. This fact alone may keep them from stopping in the middle, as they are easily distracted and lose interest quickly.

Traditionally in hammering metal, the goal in mental health has been to externalize hostility and anger and thus turn both to a constructive activity. However, in some cases, these negative emotions are sometimes increased rather than decreased through a destructive/constructive crafts (Department of the Army, 1971; Fidler, Fidler, 1954; Wilkinson, Heater, 1979).

Pediatrics

With children, using copper tooling on templates ensures a successful outcome. However, creativity is greatly reduced. For small children, simple drawing is better, as it allows for self-expression. However, older children or teens may be able to design a pattern with enough contrast to provide an interesting creative opportunity. The same precautions (i.e., self-injury) that apply to adult physically and mentally disabled clients should be observed with children and adolescents. The gross motor aspect of hammering often appeals to children. Children can be successful doing chasing by using a toothpick to make the design on copper or tin sheets. Additionally, children can do piercing with a push-pin, which requires no hammer. The large head of the push-pin allows their fingers to hold more easily than a slender implement such as a nail on a pie tin. A child using the nailing technique for piercing must coordinate both hammer and nail while trying to pierce.

Geriatrics

Again, the no-fail feature of tooling on a plastic template makes this craft attractive for therapists working with the elderly. This activity is appropriate for the diverse nursing home population (Gould, Gould, 1971). It is age appropriate, providing adult gratification with minimal cognitive requirements. With geriatric clients it is probably better to use the precut foil sheets rather than rolls of copper foil, as it decreases the steps that an elderly person must remember. This also decreases the chances of inadvertent self-injury. The elderly need special precautions because they heal more slowly. Liver of sulfur may cause clients with vision problems to complain of eye irritation. In addition, some older people may have difficulty seeing the design on the shiny metal surface.

It is often best to start clients new to crafts with this kind of simple activity/occupation; however, one danger is once elderly clients have begun to rely on a pattern, it may be difficult to break them of the copying habit (Weisburg, Wilder, 1985).

CASE STUDY

Mabel was a 78-year-old caucasian client who was admitted to the geriatric unit of a psychiatric treatment program. She was brought to the unit by her son and daughter-in-law after being referred by her internist. She appeared clearly depressed, but her psychiatrist in the hospital wanted to rule out possible dementia, as the two illnesses so often have similar symptoms. The occupational therapist was a key member of the evaluation team because he was so often able to determine whether functional deficits were truly cognitive or emotional. The occupational therapist and certified occupational therapy assistant (COTA) usually utilized the Learning/Cognitive Disabilities theories in evaluating and treating their clients.

The day of her admission, the occupational therapist performed a screening interview. Halfway through the session, her daughter-in-law joined them. She was able to add helpful information. Mabel was born and raised near the same city in which she was hospitalized. She had married her childhood sweetheart, who was a farmer, 2 days after she graduated from high school. Within 6 years, they had five children. Mabel assumed a great deal of responsibility on the farm in addition to her roles as homemaker and mother.

Involvement in the church was an important aspect of their rural community. After the children were all gone from home, she and her husband continued to farm the land. They were disappointed that one of the children had not chosen to take it over for them, but it never occurred to them to sell the farm and retire. One year ago, her husband died following several years of struggling with congestive heart disease. She had cared for him and run the farm during those years. Following his death, she had gradually started to go downhill, to be less involved in the farm operation, to avoid community and church events, and to be more dependent on her son and his wife. Recently, she had stopped taking an interest in her self-care. Her son and his wife were the only ones of her family still living nearby. A decision was made on the telephone with her other children for her to move to the nearby city to live with her son and his wife. Her condition had worsened despite the fact that she was getting more medical attention.

The following day, the occupational therapist evaluated Mabel's sensory functions, hearing, vision, smell, taste, and touch. He asked the female COTA to evaluate her on dressing and grooming and to utilize the Large Allen Cognitive Levels Test. During these evaluations, the client had repeatedly said, "I can't remember anything." She responded, "I don't know," to most questions. It appeared that she just did not want to make an effort. She had some hearing loss, especially in locating the source of sounds. Her taste and smell discrimination were somewhat diminished but still functional. Her vision was adequate when she was reminded to put on her glasses. There were no tactile deficits. She dressed and groomed herself independently but needed many prompts and encouraging remarks from the COTA. On the Allen Cognitive Levels Test she scored level 5.0, in which she corrected an error she made. The occupational therapist made the following goals with Mabel:

- To increase her self-esteem
- To increase her activity/occupation level
- To develop motivation for improved self-care

The occupational therapist asked the COTA to start Mabel out on some copper tooling.

Initially, Mabel tried to get the COTA to choose a template design so the COTA asked Mabel to choose from among three: the praying hands, the madonna, and the ballerina. She chose the praying hands. The COTA helped her tape the precut copper foil on the back of the template. Mabel started to work the impression, but by that time the first session was over. The following day she completed the tooling and filled the back with plasticine clay. The following day she applied the liver of sulfur. By the time it was dry, the session was over. During the third session she wore gloves while she polished off the black oxidation. Then she lacquered it; and at the fourth session, she put the precut cardboard frame over it. She seemed pleased with her effort despite the statement, "I would have done better 2 years ago." With the COTA's help, she hung the copper tooling in her hospital room. Mabel asked to copper tool the ballerina to give to her granddaughter.

The physician's final primary diagnosis of Mabel was depression, though he felt there was some cognitive loss as well. When she was discharged after 7 days in the hospital, Mabel told the occupational therapist and COTA that she planned to hang her praying hands in her room at her son's home, where it had been decided she would live permanently. She continued in outpatient therapy with the physician. Occasionally, she stopped to visit with the COTA and told her that at the local senior citizens' center she did another copper tooling before she decided to move on to more challenging projects in the craft room.

DISCUSSION QUESTIONS

1. Would it have been better to encourage Mabel to try a different craft for her second project?

2. Considering Mabel's sensory deficits, can you think of a craft that might have been more appropriate?

3. If you were to use copper tooling with an HIV-infected client, what would the hazards be for the client, for the therapist, or for the other clients? What precautions should be taken?

REFERENCES

Arris, R., Cordero, J., & Christiaansen, R. (1986). Occupational therapist's use of media. *Am J Occup Ther, 40*(10), 679-684.

Ayers, A. J. (1949). An analysis of crafts in the treatment of electroshock patients. *Am J Occup Ther, 3*(4), 195-198.

Department of the Army. (1951). *Occupational therapy.* Washington DC: U. S. Government Printing Office.

Department of the Army. (1971). *Craft techniques in occupational therapy.* Washington DC: U.S. Government Printing Office.

Dunton, W.R. (1945). *Prescribing occupational therapy*, 2nd ed. Springfield, IL: Charles C. Thomas.

Fidler, G. S., & Fidler, J. W. (1954). *Introduction to psychiatric occupational therapy.* New York: The MacMillan Co.

Gould, E., & Gould L. (1971). *Crafts for the elderly.* Springfield, IL: Charles C. Thomas Publisher.

Griswold, L. (1931). *Handicrafts.* Colorado Springs, CO: Outwest Printing and Stationary Company.

Johnson, C., Lobdell, K., Nesbitt, J., & Clare, M. (1996). *Therapeutic crafts: A practical approach.* Thorofare, NJ: SLACK Incorporated.

McCann, M. (1978). *Health hazards manual for artists.* New York: Foundation for the Community of Artists.

Reader's Digest. (1979). *Crafts and hobbies.* Pleasantville, NY: The Reader's Digest Association Inc.

Rich, M.K. (1960). *Handicrafts for the homebound handicapped.* Springfield, IL: Charles C. Thomas.

Titus, J. (1997.) Treatment interventions used on level II occupational therapy fieldwork. Unpublished manuscript.

Weisberg, N. & Wilder, R. (1985). *Creative arts with older adults: A sourcebook.* New York: Human Sciences Press.

Wilkinson, V. C., & Heater, S. L. (1979). *Therapeutic media and techniques of application: A guide for activities therapists.* New York: Van Nostrand Reinhold Company.

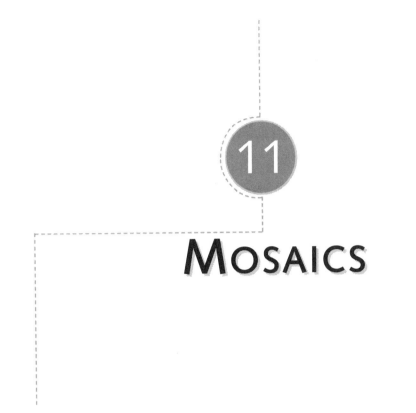

MOSAICS

INTRODUCTION

Mosaic, which is a surface decoration made of small assembled pieces, is an ancient art form probably originating in the Middle East 5000 years ago. Mosaics became very popular during the early Christian era perhaps because of its durability. Mosaics were used to make murals of sermons in pictures at a time when most people were unable to read. In those times, small pieces of colored glass, ceramic fragments, and stone were pressed into fresh plaster or concrete. The mosaic artist would have the picture and layout, colors, and shading firmly in mind. It would be necessary to do only a small area at a time and work fast (Figure 11-1). The process used today is much easier (Department of the Army, 1971; Moseley, Johnson, Koenig, 1962; *Reader's Digest*, 1979). Some other cultures in which mosaics are an important craft or art form are Greece, Egypt, Italy, Mexico, France, Thailand, Jordan, and America.

FREQUENCY OF USE

Approximately one third of clinics use mosaics once a week and another one third use mosaics somewhat less often than one time per week. As a treatment, it is most often used to improve fine motor control or to encourage self-expression (Titus, 1997).

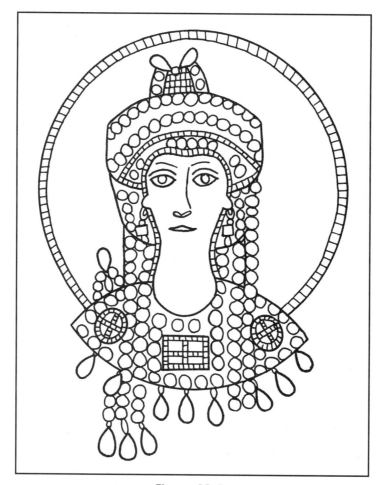

Figure 11-1.
Historical mosaic: the Empress Theodora
in San Vitale, Ravenna, Italy.

ASSESSMENTS

Mosaics require few tools, is not messy, and has the capability of assisting in assessing many functional areas such as size and color discrimination, ability to make decisions, fine motor skills, spatial awareness, ability to follow directions, and ability to organize and carry out a plan. It is included in many activity batteries. One of the earliest in occupational therapy was the Shoemyen Diagnostic Test Battery, developed between 1963 and 1967. This assessment includes clay figure modeling, sculpture carving from a composition block, finger painting, and mosaics. From one to four clients can be evaluated together. The four crafts are presented and the individual client is allowed to choose the order in which to do them. Forty-five minutes are allowed for each craft. The University of Florida developed several reporting forms for the assessment. See Table 7-1 for a profile of which crafts are used in each assessment.

The Goodman Battery, developed in 1967, starts out with the copying of a mosaic design, as it is considered to be the most structured part of the evaluation. Spontaneous drawing, figure drawing, and clay working follow this. The protocol for this assessment is strictly structured even in areas such as seating for client and therapist, placement of materials, and the pattern to copy. Cognitive and affective functioning are assessed with this battery (Hemphill, 1982).

Barbara Hemphill, who has written four books on psychiatric occupational therapy evaluation, began to develop the BH Battery in 1973. This battery has two activity components: mosaic tiling and finger painting. The tiling activity is done first, assessing skill in organizing. A layout for the materials is provided. Clients are not given design instruction other than gluing the tiles to the board however they like (Hemphill, 1982b).

The Tiled Trivet Assessment used at the Veterans Administration Medical Center in New York is part of a prevocational evaluation. This evaluation has several structured tasks: sorting screws, arranging a colored paper pattern, alphabetizing, and the Tiled Trivet Assessment. The client is asked to replicate a tile pattern using a cardboard background (Jacobs, 1991).

In the Comprehensive Assessment Process for assessment of clients in a group, mosaics are used in the first of three 50-minute sessions. The client can choose from four colors to complete a mosaic board design. At the second session, there are six choices for colored grout. The behaviors assessed have to do with interpersonal interactions, work skills, self-concept, self-knowledge, and leisure skills. Other activities in this assessment are magazine collage, a group mural, or a hypothetical group problem-solving session about landing on the moon. The group chooses one of these three activities to do at the third session. Documentation is done on a check-off sheet (Hemphill, 1982a).

The Perkins Tile Task, for use in psychiatry, was presented at the 1986 Great Southern Occupational Therapy Conference in Charleston, SC, by Vicki Perkins, OTR. Quantitative research, number of tiles used, amount of board surface covered, and tile placement were related to diagnostic groups (Perkins, 1986).

The Nedra Gillette Battery is a purely projective test that was developed in the 1960s. It has three activities, each with a different purpose: watercolor as an unstructured task, mosaic as the structured test, and carving a plaster vermiculite composite block as the resistive test. A scoring scale of behavior traits was used (Gillette, 1989).

The Neuropsychiatric Institute (NPI) Interest Checklist includes mosaics among its 80 activities. Clients are asked to complete the questionnaire about the level of their interest in the various activities. A discussion of the completed checklist between client and therapist aims to assess past, present, and possible future leisure choices (Matsutsuya, 1969).

TREATMENT WITH MOSAICS

Perhaps the attraction of this craft for today's therapist is that mosaics fit the current short hospital stays of many clients. Tile trivets, which come in a variety of shapes, are probably the most common mosaic project. The trivet frames are metal or plywood shapes into which the mosaic is set. A 6-inch square size is often used. The metal trivets purchased through craft suppliers have a masonite board on which to mount the tile. Some clinics simply give a 6 x 6-inch. board cut in the clinic for the clients. If they finish their tile project, it is then mounted in the trivet frame. In this manner, the waste that occurs when clients do not finish their project before being discharged is diminished.

In long-term facilities, residents can attempt more challenging mosaic projects such as table tops, jewelry boxes, trays, or picture frames. Another traditional mosaic-like process is using various colors and shapes of dried peas, beans, and pasta to cover shapes and spaces to make a picture (*Better Homes and Gardens*, 1966; Janitch, 1973). These make nice kitchen decorations.

Supplies

For the usual 6 x 6-inch tile trivet, the following supplies and tools are needed. Most supplies and tools will need to be purchased from craft vendors; however, tiles may be purchased more inexpensively at local tile stores that sell tiles for kitchens and bathrooms.
- Paper and pencil for making the design
- An assortment of ceramic tiles in various shapes, sizes, and colors
- A 6 x 6-inch, 1/8-inch masonite board
- Tile cement or white glue
- Grout
- Grout coloring (optional)
- Water or grout additive
- Grout sealer or liquid floor wax
- Paper towels

Tools

- Bowl for mixing
- Ruler for measuring spaces
- Spoon
- Spatula
- Tile nippers
- Sponge

Process

1. Show the client a sample of a finished trivet.
2. Have the client plan his or her own design and choose his or her tile

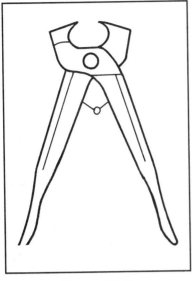

Figure 11-2.
Tile nippers.

colors. The tiles can be arranged and rearranged to fit the space until a satifactory design is chosen.

3. If tiles need to be cut to fit, the client should put on goggles before cutting with the tile nippers (Figure 11-2). If the client cuts the tiles inside a paper bag, others are also protected from flying fragments.

4. Glue the pieces down individually. Remove two at a time from the design. This allows enough working space to apply one of the two individual tiles to the board without disturbing or losing the entire design. Before gluing the second tile, remove a third to provide working space. Allow space of 1/16 to 1/8-inch between the tiles. Use a ruler as a guide if necessary. This space is wide enough for the grout to be applied between the tiles. Some suggest standing a nickel or dime between tiles to space them properly.

5. Continue gluing until the design is completed. Allow the glue to dry.

6. Mix the grout according to package directions. The powdered grout and water or grout additive mixture should be the consistency of heavy cream.

7. The grout mixture is poured or scraped with the spatula onto the tiles. Use the spatula, fingers, sponge, or damp paper towels to push the grout into all the crevices. Be sure to grout the board all the way to the edge. Tap the tile to allow air bubbles to escape; this prevents holes and cracks.

8. Lightly rub the excess grout off the tiles, being careful not to rub it out of the cracks.

9. Allow grout to dry slowly overnight. Place a damp cloth or paper towel over it. If cracks appear, mix another batch of grout and apply it into the cracks.

10. When the grout is completely dry, rub any remaining grout film off the tiles.

11. Fit the tiled board into the trivet frame.

12. Apply the grout sealer. Liquid floor wax can be used as a grout sealer (Department of the Army, 1971; Moseley, Johnson, Koenig, 1962; *Reader's Digest*, 1979; VanZandt, 1973).

MAIN THERAPEUTIC APPLICATIONS

Physical Dysfunction

For the most part, physically disabled clients' fine motor coordination can be addressed through the making of mosaics. Picking up the tiles can improve pinch. Gripping the tile nippers can be used to strengthen cylindrical grasp. The special aspects of planning and arranging the design can be important areas for those clients with brain trauma such as head injury or cerebrovascular accident (Department of the Army, 1971; Overs, O'Conner, Demarco, 1974). Mosaics may be done by bed patients and those in isolation up to the point of mixing and applying grout. That process is best done near a sink that has a clay or plaster trap to prevent the grout from clogging the drain. For bed-bound or ward-bound clients, the therapist might want to take the project to the clinic and do the grouting for them. For the one-handed client, gluing the tile down may make this craft too difficult and frustrating. Mixing the grout and water may cause dust in the air, which would be contraindicated for respiratory clients.

Mental Health

Mosaics offer opportunities to work on problems that affect many mental health clients: attention span, concentration, planning, spatial relationship, sequencing, and fine motor control. This may be why mosaics are so often used in psychiatric occupational therapy assessments. Even very low-functioning clients can achieve a good product outcome with mosaics. By increasing the tile color, shape choice, size, and complexity of the project, it is possible to grade mosaics from very easy to difficult.

Pediatrics

Pediatric clients are often working to improve fine motor performance. Mosaics provide an excellent opportunity to practice this skill. The time required to glue all the tiles frequently exceeds the attention span of many children. Gluing may need to be done in several sessions. Another inexpensive possibility with children is to use seeds and beans. Simply cover each section with glue and scatter the seeds on that section. Shake off the excess onto a newspaper and pour the excess back into the seed container. This speeds up the process for children's shorter attention spans. Another adaptation for children is paper mosaics. A variety of shapes, sizes, and colors of construction paper are used to make a design that can be glued to cardboard or paper. Girls sometimes enjoy sedentary mosaic activity more than boys.

Geriatrics

Adaptation of mosaics for the elderly may include using the 3/4-inch tiles rather than the 3/8-inch size. This increases the tiles' visibility and the ease with which they are handled. The therapist may choose highly contrasting colors, as these also make them more visible. If white or light tiles are glued on the dark brown masonite, they show up well. Mosaic materials are usually not breakable. This is beneficial since many elderly clients have poor balance, which makes it difficult for them to walk and get in and out of chairs, which may cause them to possibly drop things. They may lack the grip strength to use the tile nippers. The trivet project usually takes not longer than three sessions, thus sustaining their interest. This simple, yet attractive, craft can be appealing to the elderly, as its rich history may make it seem like a prestigious craft and thus age appropriate.

CASE STUDY

Michael is a 69-year-old Lebanese immigrant. He grew up in Beirut in a Christian family. After attending a school run by missionaries, he went to a university in France to study architecture. World War II broke out while he was in France. He joined the French Army, was captured and spent several years as a prisoner of war. After the war, he returned to Beirut and completed his architectural studies at the American University. Michael joined an architectural company and began to develop a name for himself locally as a restoration specialist for old buildings. In 1950, his family assisted him in arranging a marriage with a second cousin. The couple had four children during the next 10 years.

He and his wife were very concerned about their children's education. They sacrificed luxuries to send their children to private schools and the university. As the three older children finished college, they left the parental home. The eldest, a girl, followed in her father's footsteps and went to France to study medicine. The second eldest, a male, took a job working in Saudi Arabia. The next boy was accepted as a student at the University of Oklahoma and went to the United States, leaving only the youngest daughter at home. The three children living in other countries returned home for yearly visits.

When Israel invaded Lebanon, Michael and his wife and daughter remained in their home, which Michael had built gradually in stages over the years in the Christian section of Beirut. As the war progressed and the bombing came closer, the three older children began to press their parents to emigrate. In 1984, Michael's wife died of a heart attack during a particularly close and heavy bomb attack. At last, he was persuaded to emigrate to the United States, where his youngest son lived with his American wife.

He and the youngest daughter, who was 25 years old, were crowded into this American home. Michael had to share a room with his grandson.

Shortly after his arrival, he began to have angina. The physician who examined him found him to be a good candidate for open heart surgery for coronary artery disease. This was performed in 1985. In the years following this surgery, Michael became very fearful and depressed. He became a cardiac cripple, refusing to do the exercises advised by his physician. He just sat on the sofa in front of the television. He then developed a sleep disturbance, sleep apnea. The combination of the sleep problem with the inactivity caused him to become increasingly depressed and cranky. His son's family found him to be very disturbing to their family life. His daughter, who spoke very little English, was of little help in coping with her father. When he began to refuse to eat, his condition rapidly deteriorated.

Finally, he had a panic attack, fearing he was dying. His son called an ambulance, and he was taken to the emergency department. After a triage screening, it was decided he needed further observation for his disorientation, but not for his heart. He was admitted to the hospital's geropsychiatric rehabilitation unit. His physician consulted with the psychiatrist on the unit, and they gave him a diagnosis of organic anxiety syndrome with depression and sleep apnea. Both physicians advised gradually increasing his activity level while they ran further tests.

The occupational therapist evaluated Michael using a geriatric sensory screening and the Goodman Battery. The theories subscribed to by this therapist were the Lifestyle/Adaptive Performance and the Learning/Cognitive Disabilities models. The tests she chose fit these models. On the mosaic tile task, Michael surprised the therapist by completing the replication of the tile sample quickly and accurately. He mentioned that some of the buildings he had restored in Beirut had had mosaic floor tiles. His spontaneous drawing was a sketch of one of the buildings Michael remembered working on years ago. In the human figure drawings, he drew a typical Middle Eastern workman holding a shovel and wearing the traditional Arab headdress. He said he was too tired to finish the clay portion of the test that day, so it was postponed. His physicians at this time discovered he had an obstructed airway.

Surgery was performed to remove the obstruction. The occupational therapist went to visit him in the recovery room. When he returned to the geropsychiatric rehabilitation unit the next day, she showed him some books on mosaics that she had checked out of the public library. She set a bookrack up for him on his bedside table and stayed with him for half an hour while he looked at and discussed the books. He never finished the clay portion of the Goodman Battery because he became involved in creating a mosaic table top to give to his daughter-in-law. As he began to eat and sleep better and to draw his mosaic design and choose his tiles, his depression began to lift and the dementia seemed to clear. Part of his discharge plan included returning three times per week for the outpatient program. He completed the mosaic design but was unable to finish putting on the legs before his discharge from the outpatient program. Before his discharge, the certified occupational therapy assistant took Michael to a local senior center to orient him with resources for senior citizens. Initially, he was reluctant and shy, as he was the only male with 15 women at the center.

A craft room had supervision 6 hours per day. The center activity director assured Michael that there were several other men who attended as well. He appeared pleased and mildly excited by the arts and crafts area and the prospect of finishing his table.

DISCUSSION QUESTIONS

1. Would one of the other assessment batteries have been a better choice for Michael? Why?
2. If Michael had been dissatisfied with the ceramic mosaic tiles available to him in the occupational therapy clinic, what could the therapist have done to get glass tiles, which were satisfactory to him? Where might a therapist go to find glass tiles that are seldom used now, rather than the ceramic tiles she had available?
3. What precautions could be necessary for a client who just had an airway obstruction removed?

REFERENCES

Better Homes and Gardens. (1966). *Stitchery and crafts.* New York: Meredith Press.

Department of the Army. (1971). *Craft techniques in occupational therapy.* Washington D.C.: U.S. Government Printing Office.

Gillette, N. (July 2, 1989). Personal communication—telephone interview and letter regarding Nedra Gillette's Battery. Birmingham, AL.

Hemphill, B. J. (1982a). *The evaluative process in psychiatric occupational therapy.* Thorofare, NJ: SLACK Incorporated.

Hemphill, B.J. (1982b). *Training manual for the BH battery.* Thorofare, NJ: SLACK Incorporated.

Jacobs, K. (1991). *Occupational therapy: Work-related programs and assessments* (2nd ed.). Boston: Little, Brown and Company.

Janitch, V. (1973). *Country crafts.* New York: Viking Press.

Matsutsuya, J. S. (1969). The interest checklist. *Am J Occup Ther, 23*(4),323-328.

Moseley, S., Johnson, P., & Koenig, H. (1962). *Crafts design.* Belmont, CA: Wadsworth.

Overs, R. P., O'Conner, E., & Demarco, B. (1974). *Avocational activities for the handicapped.* Springfield, IL: Charles C. Thomas.

Perkins, V. J. (1986). Quantitative assessment of a mosaic tile task. Abstracts of the Fourth Annual Meeting. The Great Southern Occupational Therapy Conference. Charleston, SC.

Reader's Digest. (1979). *Crafts and hobbies.* Pleasantville, NY: Reader's Digest Association, Inc.

Titus, J. (1997). Treatment interventions used on level II occupational therapy fieldwork. Unpublished manuscript.

VanZandt, V. (1973). *Crafts for fun and profit.* London: Aldus Books.

CERAMICS

INTRODUCTION

The ancient craft of ceramics involves simply shaping clay (an especially plastic earth), allowing it to dry, and then baking it at a high temperature for a long period of time. Ceramics may be one of our oldest crafts developed after leatherworking and woodworking. We know humans have been shaping clay and baking it for 10,000 years. In fact, the durability of pottery fragments have made it possible for archeologists to learn much about prehistoric humans. On the other hand, ceramics break, so intact ancient pieces are rare. These characteristics, brittleness yet durability, remain despite our advanced technology in other areas (Budworth, 1970; Marmer, 1997).

Ceramics is an encompassing term that includes pottery, ceramic sculpture, ceramic tiles used in kitchens and bathrooms, ceramic building blocks and decorative facades for buildings, beads, and jewelry, as well as the ceramic tiles used to protect the bodies of space shuttles. The scope of this book includes only a minute part of what are called ceramics—only those objects usually made by clients working with occupational therapists: smaller pots, sculptures, and jewelry. New materials and instruction books for their use appear with regularity, allowing for creative uses of clay-like materials without the inconvenience of firing a kiln (Dierks, 1994).

FREQUENCY OF USE

One quarter to one third of therapists use ceramics in their clinical practice. The most frequently used types are slip-molded greenware and ceramic sculpture. Few clinics and therapists are able to afford the time and energy expenditure to use the potter's wheel. However, since ceramics techniques are similar to those of a variety of less durable shaping and sculpting materials, it is best to present these basic craft techniques, which can be adapted to the other materials.

ASSESSMENTS

Standardized occupational therapy assessments that use clay as part of a complete evaluation are the Goodman Battery, the Shoemyen Battery, the Azima Battery, Carolyn Owens Activity Battery, Gillette's Battery, Nelson Clark's Clay Test, Androes, Dreyfus and Bloesch Diagnostic Occupational Therapy Test Battery, Gross Activity Battery, and O'Kane Diagnostic Battery. These are all evaluations used with psychiatric clients. In most of them, the client is asked to use the provided clay to make something. However, the Shoemyen Battery specifically asks the client to model a human figure (Hemphill, 1982). Each of these evaluations includes the projective clay sculpture as part of a battery of activities. Even Clark's Clay Test is part of the Clark Battery (Moyer, 1983). Clay is included because it is a part of natural human development to attempt to shape. Scribbling and drawing have similar developmental sequences. Initially, the child smears, feels, and squeezes clay, and then molds shapes (Harris, 1963; O'Kane, 1968). Clay is viewed as the most unstructured of all projective assessments because of the effort needed to control it. Its plastic quality allows a client to make a mistake and reverse it. The aspects of clay that allow a client to express many emotions, ideas, and qualities also cause difficulty for those with perceptual dysfunction (Hemphill, 1982). For purposes of construction, three-dimensional media are more difficult to conceptualize than two-dimensional media (Turoff, 1949).

Supplies

It is possible to use ceramics in a room or section off the occupational therapy clinic following safety guidelines for kiln wiring and venting. Such specifications are usually available through the safety officer of your hospital or clinic, or the local ceramics store. The sink for ceramics needs to have a clay sediment trap in the drainpipe to allow clay residue to be easily removed and thus avoid costly plumbing bills. The following supplies and equipment are sufficient for most clinic ceramics and for the techniques discussed in this book, although more sophisticated materials and techniques are available.

- Ready-mixed clay
- Ready-mixed slip
- Ready-mixed glazes
- Bisque stains and spray
- Fine-grain sponges
- Pyrometric cones
- Kiln wash
- Underglazes

TOOLS AND EQUIPMENT

- Covered plastic clay storage container
- Storage shelves
- Kiln
- Kiln furniture
- Stilts
- Canvas-covered boards
- Clay pull (cutting wire)
- Fettling knife
- Sgraffito/cleaning tool
- Needle tool
- Wire-loop tool
- Rolling pin
- Plaster or masonite bats
- Slip molds
- Slip strainer
- Mold straps
- Sink
- Plastic water bowls
- Glaze brushes

Process

Most therapists buy ready-ground and mixed clay, as the preparation of unground and unmixed clay is difficult and requires extensive costly machinery. Clay is usually purchased in 25-pound plastic bags that measure approximately 14 x 5 x 5 inches. Clay comes in a variety of grays, browns, and reds. Clay can have grog added, which is previously fired clay ground up like sand. This adds strength to the clay but is contraindicated for many clients, as it can be abrasive to the hands. Different clays may fire at different temperatures, however, most occupational therapists simplify their ceramics operation by firing at only one or two temperatures, usually between 1800° and 2000°F or between 980° and 1100°C.

The first step in preparing the ready-mixed clay is to cut and form it into usable 3- to 4-inch diameter pieces. This is most easily accomplished

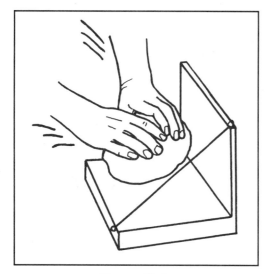

Figure 12-1.
Wedging on a wedging board.

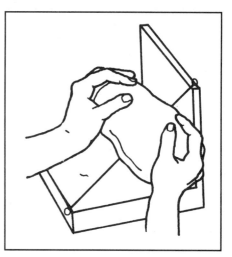

Figure 12-2.
Cutting clay on the wire.

by using the clay pull, which is a tool one can easily make by cutting a 20-inch length of thin wire or nylon fishing line and tying each end to a large button or bead.

The clay pull is grasped at each end and wound around the fingers until it is quite close to the clay. The line is laid across the block and pressed straight down through the clay until the proper size piece can be pulled off. This piece is then wedged. Professional ceramicists wedge clay in a kneading pattern, but in occupational therapy the most common method is to throw the clay onto a wedging board, as shown in the illustration (Figure 12-1). The purpose of wedging is to redistribute the moisture equally to make the clay softer and easier to handle and to get rid of any air pockets that could possibly cause the piece to explode in the kiln when the heated air expands during firing. The wedged clay is then cut on a wire (Figure 12-2) or with the clay pull to assure that no air pockets remain (Figure 12-3). It is then rewedged before using.

There are six basic methods of forming ceramics in occupational therapy. They are described and illustrated sequentially below from the easiest technique (pinch pots) to the most difficult and exacting (the potter's wheel).

Pinch Pot

PROCESS

1. Form the clay into a ball.
2. Stick the thumb into the top of the ball. This makes the first opening.
3. With the thumb of the dominant hand on the inside and fingers on the outside, begin to press gently out with the thumb, moving the

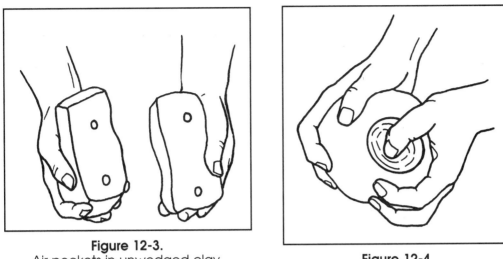

Figure 12-3.
Air pockets in unwedged clay.

Figure 12-4.
Pinch pot.

form either clockwise or counter clockwise while keeping the piece supported with the nondominant hand (Figure 12-4). Continue to move the beginning vessel in this fashion until the walls and bottom are uniformly 1/2-inch thick or less. If small cracks appear on the edge near the opening, just pinch them together.

4. Set the pot on a canvas-covered board and, using both hands, smooth the walls. Do not use water to smooth the walls at this point, as it will weaken them.

5. Set the pot aside to dry on a mesh shelf or grate so air can reach all surfaces.

6. After it is leather hard, or the hardness of good shoe leather, smooth the pot with a damp, fine-grain sponge. At this stage, carve or incise the surface for decoration.

The length of the drying process depends on the temperature, humidity, and movement of the air. Most hospitals have a fairly dry atmosphere. Therapists will need to experiment to find how long it takes a piece to become bone dry, which has occurred when the piece is not cool to the touch, but feels like room temperature. Then the piece will be ready to bisque fire—a process to be described later.

Slab Building

Slab construction is the next most complicated process.

PROCESS

1. On a canvas-covered board, roll the wedged clay with a rolling pin to an even thickness of 1/2 to 1/4 inch.

2. Lay a previously made paper pattern on the clay. Cut around the

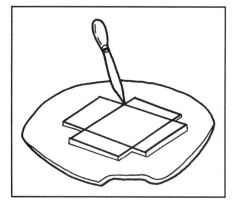

Figure 12-5.
Cutting around a paper pattern
with a fettling knife.

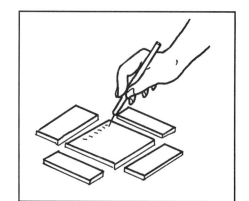

Figure 12-6.
Crosshatching with a clay needle.

pattern with a fettling knife (Figure 12-5), which is a special clay tool for cutting.

3. After a short time in which the pieces are allowed to slightly stiffen, join the pieces in the following manner: lift the base off the canvas and place it on a plaster bat.

4. Incise or score all the edges that are to be joined by using a tool called a needle, which is a wooden cylinder handle with a 1 1/2-inch pin stuck into the end (Figure 12-6). The incising should be in a crosshatch manner. Each seam will have two crosshatch edges.

5. Moisten both edges with a finger before pressing them together. This moisture goes into the incisions and makes a natural slip. Slip is a liquid clay that is used for a variety of purposes, one of which will be described later. In slab building, one must be careful not to allow the clay to become too wet, as that weakens the structure.

6. Strengthen the joints by pressing a coil of clay on the interior surface and smoothing it into the walls.

7. Then set the piece aside until it is leather hard, when it can be decorated by sgraffito, textured with a comb, or impressions with buttons or other small objects can be made.

Slab building may offer the most variety of all techniques in ceramics. Napkin rings can be constructed with one simple joint. A simple slab scored on the bottom to prevent warping and decorated with surface designs makes an attractive trivet. A draped slab can be made by laying a trimmed clay slab over another object to dry. Buttons, buckles, and windchime parts can all be cut from a plain slab.

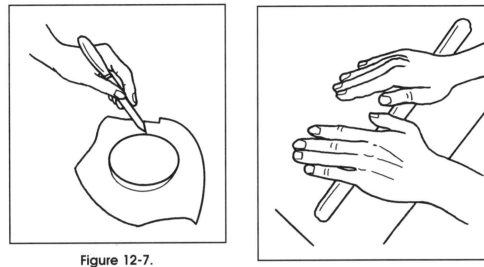

Figure 12-7.
Cutting a round base
for a coil pot.

Figure 12-8.
Coils being made.

Coil Building

Coil building is an elaboration of the slab-building technique.

PROCESS

1. Make a round or oval base slab (Figure 12-7).
2. Score or incise the edge where the coil will be placed.
3. Make the coils by rolling the piece back and forth with both hands on the canvas-covered board (Figure 12-8).
4. Wet the scored edge and lay the coil on it.
5. Press it lightly to bond the two pieces.
6. Lightly moisten the top of the coil; lay another coil on this seam and lightly press.
7. Continue this process until the desired height is reached. If the pot is to curve outward, set the coil a little to the outside of the one below it. If it is to curve inward, place the coil a little toward the inside top surface of the preceding coil.
8. When the desired shape and size are reached, smooth the sides. Many people like the look of coil pots and, consequently, do nothing to change the surface. It is possible to use coils in making the base, but these are never quite as strong as a slab base. In each slip-bonded joint lies the potential for weakness and possible cracking.
9. Another easy coil method, especially for wide, low bowls that have the potential to collapse from their own weight while damp, is to select a ready-made bowl, line it with plastic wrap, lay the slab for the base in the bottom of the bowl, then lay the coils up the sides

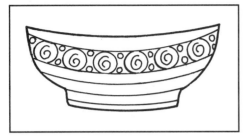

Figure 12-9.
A bowl with coil design.

of the bowl. A design can be made with the coils (Figure 12-9). The plastic wrap leaves minimal marks.

10. Coils should be smoothed on the inside of the bowl to fasten them together, for neatness and easy washability.

11. The coiled bowl should be left inside the ready-made bowl until it is leather hard, then it can be lifted out.

Sculpture

Sculpture in occupational therapy is often an activity in which the therapist offers very little instruction or direction to the client. Sculpture incorporates the techniques used to make pinch pots, slab containers, and coil vessels, as well as techniques not previously mentioned. One such technique involves using a piece of clay and hollowing the center out by using a wire loop tool to systematically cut away pieces of clay from the middle or inside of a bulky sculpture. This prevents an explosion, as sculptures with thick walls are prone to blow up in the kiln. Another technique is to use a paper core or substructure and form the clay sculpture around it. The paper core, which supports the sculpture's walls and keeps it from collapsing in on itself, will burn away in the kiln, leaving a hollow sculpture. Professional sculptors use other techniques in building larger, more complex figures, but they are too involved for most clinical situations. Children often assemble parts when making a sculpture, for example, sticking a head, arms, and legs to a torso to make a person. These parts often break off in handling or firing unless the child uses the correct technique for joining parts.

Slip Casting

Slip casting is the process of pouring liquid clay into a preformed plaster mold and allowing the clay to accumulate as a layer on the plaster wall before pouring out the remaining liquid clay. Slip casting is often used by many therapists because chances of a successful product are good, which will please the client and increase self-esteem.

Mold making is a complex process requiring skills beyond the scope of this book. Many moderately priced molds are available at local ceramic hobby stores.

PROCESS

1. First check the slip-casting molds for cleanliness and gently wipe

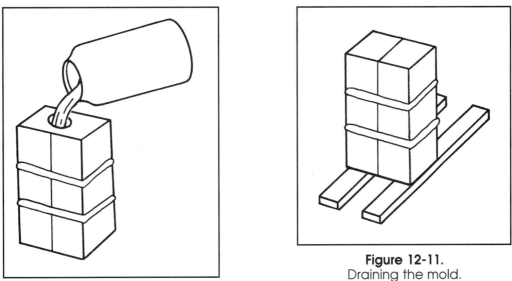

Figure 12-10.
Pouring slip into a mold.

Figure 12-11.
Draining the mold.

them out with a damp sponge or fine bristle paint brush, if necessary, to remove old clay.

2. Fit the mold sections together and fasten them tightly with mold straps or giant rubber bands.

3. Mix and strain the slip to remove any lumps.

4. Pour the slip into the mold pour spout (Figure 12-10) to the top.

5. As the plaster absorbs moisture from the slip, it will sink down in the pour spout. It is necessary to check the mold every few minutes and refill it to the top.

6. When the thickness of the solid clay near the plaster becomes approximately 1/4 inch, pour out the remainder of the slip by turning the mold over to drain (Figure 12-11). This slip can be saved and reused if stored properly in an airtight container.

7. After approximately half an hour, turn the mold upright and carefully remove one half of the mold.

8. Cut off the excess clay in the pour spout. The piece can remain in the half mold until it becomes leather hard. It will then easily come out of the mold because in drying, it will shrink away from the plaster (Figure 12-12).

9. If the slip casting has textured walls, allow it to dry before cleaning the seams with a sgraffito/cleaning tool. If the slip cast has no texture or detail, the seam can be removed at the leather-hard stage with a fine-grain sponge. There are a variety of other molds, press molds, and drape molds that can also be used with regular

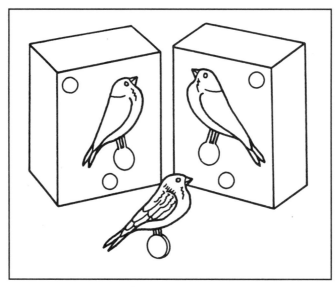

Figure 12-12.
Removing a piece from the mold.

clay instead of slip. These molds are usually one piece into which clay is pressed or draped and removed when leather hard.

Pottery Wheel

Throwing on the potter's wheel is one of the most sophisticated ceramic techniques. Consequently, few clinics use it because of the skill required for a client to successfully create an object. Only the most basic steps will be given here. Students of ceramics wishing for more information will find a variety of source books (Turoff, 1949; Department of the Army, 1971; Hamilton, 1974; Nelson, 1966; Wettlaufer, Wettlaufer, 1976).

PROCESS

1. Experiment with the foot pedal or switch to determine how much pressure or power is required to achieve the desired speed.
2. Affix a bat on the center of the wheel. A bowl of water and a sponge should be nearby.
3. Very slightly dampen the bat.
4. Place a ball of wedged clay the size of an orange onto the center of the bat (Figure 12-13).
5. Start the wheel slowly and check with a finger to be sure the ball is in the center of the wheel. If it is not, stop the wheel and reposition the clay. Repeat this until the ball is as close as possible to the center. Then with the wheel stopped, press it down to fasten it to the bat.
6. The clay must be kept "slippery" wet so that it slips through the hands. The potter needs to constantly reapply water to the surface.

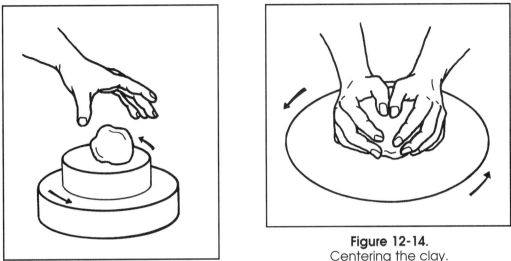

Figure 12-13.
Tossing clay onto the
center of the bat.

Figure 12-14.
Centering the clay.

The wheel should always be moving before the hands touch the clay and be kept moving after the hands have been gently removed from the clay. Begin to spin the wheel and press the palms of both hands down and around the base of the clay to center it (Figure 12-14). Keeping the forearms braced on the thighs helps stabilize the hands and wrists. The basic principle to remember is that force to the clay should be transmitted through pressure from the large bones of the arm and wrist so the muscles don't cramp and tire, and because it works better.

7. Coning is the next step in which the clay is actually mixed by pressing to raise it to a cone shape, then steadily pressing down on the top of the cone with the right hand while supporting the clay with the left hand (Figure 12-15). This is all done with the palms of the hands, not the fingers. In occupational therapy, clients are encouraged to practice joint protection using large muscles and joints rather than putting stress on the more vulnerable small joints and tendons. Advanced potters repeat the coning process several times before the next step (Figure 12-16). Beginners may omit coning and move immediately to step 8.

8. Open the clay. This is achieved by pressing the right thumb into the middle of the centered clay as the wheel continues to move (Figure 12-17). The thumb is pressed to a depth that leaves about 1 inch of clay between the thumb and bat. Then place both thumbs in the hole and begin to slowly and gently widen it until the floor of the pot is the desired width.

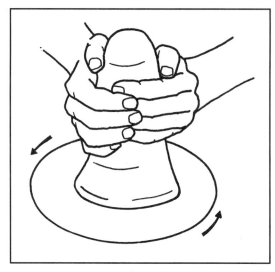

Figure 12-15.
Coning the clay.

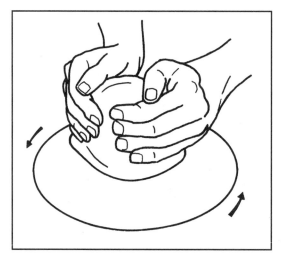

Figure 12-16.
Pressing down on clay in
preparation for reconing.

9. Next, raise the walls by interlocking the thumbs and placing the
fingers of the left hand inside the hole and the right on the outside.
As the wheel revolves, apply gentle pressure while pulling up at the
same time. Keeping the elbows in and at the side or with the forearms on the thighs improves control. Repeat this motion until the
desired height is reached. For beginners, objects of 6 inches in
height and 4 inches in diameter are all that should be attempted.
Simple cylinders or bowls are adequate for most clients. Shaping
the clay into other than a cylindrical shape or small bowl takes
skill and practice.

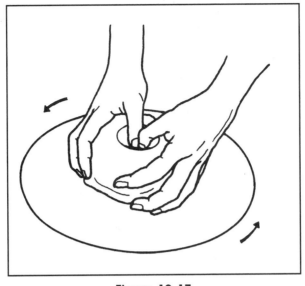

Figure 12-17.
Opening up the clay.

10. When the pot is fully formed, use a damp sponge to smooth the inside of the pot and absorb excess water, which could weaken the walls.
11. Level the top of the vessel by placing the needle tool through the wall 1/2 to 1/4 inch below the top while the wheel is slowly turning and then trimming away this clay until the top edge is even. Then smooth the rim with wet fingers or a sponge while the wheel is turning.
12. Loosen the vessel by pulling the clay along the surface between the pot and the masonite bat once. This is not necessary with plaster bats.
13. Then set the pot aside on the bat until it is leather hard.
14. Lift the pot off the bat.
15. Turn it upside down, center it on the wheel, and stabilize it with three pieces of fresh clay. This process, called turning, involves trimming off the excess clay at the base.
16. Make concentric circles with the needle tool while the wheel turns (Figure 12-18). This shows the potter where the clay is too thick so it may be trimmed, making the walls of the pot equally thick throughout.
17. Then, pare the excess clay by using cutting tools. Take the pot off the bat.
18. Texture or incise the walls for decoration and allow the pot to dry.

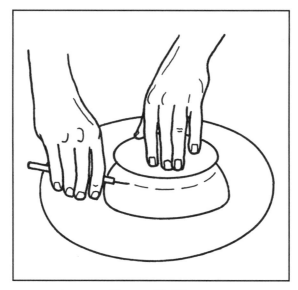

Figure 12-18.
Trimming the pot with the needle tool.

FIRING THE KILN

Each kiln comes with a firing manual that gives a timing guide and loading directions. Most clinic firing is between the pyrometric cone range of 07 to 03. The first firing is called the bisque firing, which causes the clay to harden enough so that it will not disintegrate if it becomes wet. For clients, all clay should be bisque fired to make the piece more durable before glaze is applied.

Kiln firing by gas may expose the individual doing the firing to carbon monoxide, which can cause brain injury, so precautions for ventilation are particularly important (Anonymous, 1986).

Glazes

Glazes in clinics are almost always ready-mixed, as some of the ingredients when in the dry state are hazardous to health. Commercial glazes have specific directions for application and firing temperature on the label. Glazes should dry at least 6 hours before firing.

UNDERGLAZES

Underglaze is another kind of surface decoration. It can be brushed, sponged, spattered, or sprayed onto bisqueware. Look at the label for application and firing instructions. The piece must be fired again before applying clear or semitransparent overglaze. Underglazed pieces need an overglaze and a third firing to give a water impermeable surface. Underglaze offers opportunities for experimentation, such as brushing the underglaze into incisions on the surface to emphasize them or brushing the underglaze over a textured surface and rubbing away some of the glaze to emphasize the texture. Ceramic hobbyists often brush underglaze onto greenware, but greenware is usually too fragile for most sick people to handle with the delicacy required. It is necessary to bisque fire everything in the clinic before glazing or underglazing.

BISQUE STAINS

For purely decorative pieces such as figurines and some kinds of jewelry, bisque stains can be painted on the surface. These stains, which are unfired, are not moisture resistant and cannot be used in any container that may hold liquids. However, they have some qualities that make them useful in the clinic.

They do not require as much time or as many processes as traditional glazes. They should be applied over gray clay, which becomes white after firing, as the color will be clearer than over red or brown clay (Marmer, 1997). Stains are applied in much the same way as liquid tempra paints; and like tempra colors, they need to have a protective finish over them. Most commonly, a spray sealer is used. This kind of sealer needs to be applied where there is adequate ventilation, preferably outdoors. In some situations, the client can apply the stain to the bisqueware and the therapist will then apply the lacquer sealer for the client. Be careful to avoid setting the piece with those to be fired, as they may be hard to tell apart at firing time.

The last firing is the glaze firing. Glazed pieces should be set on stilts and placed so there is at least 1/2 an inch between each piece and the walls. This allows air to circulate, thus avoiding spotty glazes. Clients, like many ceramicists, have difficulty waiting the length of time required for proper kiln cooling. A rule of thumb is to let the kiln cool twice as long as it took to fire it to full temperature. This will avoid having glazes craze and crackle from cooling too fast.

MAIN THERAPEUTIC APPLICATIONS

Physical Dysfunction

In the past, before the age of therapy putty (a moldable plastic or silicone substance), ceramic clay was used to achieve all the same benefits for which that expensive medium is now used. Squeezing, pushing, pinching, patting, rolling, smoothing, and manipulating clay can achieve almost any wrist, hand, or finger movement desired. Working with clay strengthens the upper extremities and can easily be graded from delicate manipulations such as patting, to pushing, pressing, and throwing clay during wedging, or wedging by kneading. Wedging can achieve shoulder flexion and extension. Rolling the clay uses the abdominals, elbow extensors, and flexors. The therapist must be careful that the table and chair are the proper height to achieve the desired movement. Positioning of the project will define which muscles are used. The therapist needs to think through exactly which motions are desired and raise or lower the project, place it closer or farther or to the side of the client to achieve the desired movement. Fine motor control and coordination can be enhanced by scoring the clay in slab or coil building, or applying surface decorative techniques such as sgraffito or painting with underglazes.

Theoretically, the kick wheel should be good for strengthening knee extensors, but practically, throwing a pot on the wheel requires so much concentration and skill that it is difficult to coordinate the upper extremity with the needs of a healing lower extremity. Clay can be used with bedside clients, as it is noise free if the clay is already wedged. Damp clay is nontoxic and easily washable. It can be worked with or without tools. All these attributes make it a good medium to carry into the room of a client confined for infectious disease. It is less expensive than therapy putty and can be left in the client's room. A masonite square covered with paper can be used as a work surface. If an infectious client completes a project for firing, the whole working surface with clay on top can be put into a plastic bag to be carried to the kiln. All infectious agents will be killed in firing. The paper should be bagged for disposal like all other infection-controlled materials. The masonite can be sterilized by washing with antibacterial soap.

Clay is particularly suited for use with the blind and partially sighted because of its tactile qualities. The blind person can feel a sample and use that shape to formulate an idea to work toward. One-handed clients can succeed at coil-built pots if the therapist cuts a base. Both using the rolling pin and rolling coils can cause the client to use a weak hand to assist or stabilize in the movement. Additionally, these two movements require the client to work on trunk control, which is a problem for many stroke clients. For clients with poor coordination, the draped slab method may achieve the best results.

Burn patients with completely healed wounds can work on decreasing contractures by working with clay. Because their skin is so tender and clay dries it out, each session with clay should be followed by applying hand lotion.

Conditions in which ceramics are contraindicated are in clients whose hands have open wounds, because of the possibility of infection or further damage to the wounded surface; arthritic joints can be further damaged by too much force since many ceramic techniques can stress joints; clients with circulation problems, as with diabetes, should not participate as even smooth clay can abrade the skin surface; and clients with nerve deficits can injure their hands without feeling it (Turoff, 1949; Department of the Army, 1971; Hamill, Oliver, 1989; Wilkinson, Heater, 1979).

Mental Health

The opportunity for expression of thought and mood are perhaps the most beneficial aspects of clay for psychiatric clients. Listed earlier in this chapter are several psychiatric occupational therapy evaluations that use clay. The clay project can demonstrate cognitive deficits such as confusion, inability to follow instructions, as well as a depressed mood or bizarre thoughts. For clients with cognitive deficits, having a variety of samples for them to examine assists in conceptualizing the clay process. While schizophrenics may have difficulty with the formlessness of a pinch pot or clay sculpture, both wedging and rolling slabs or coils can achieve the shoulder external rotation and elbow extension that are so often deficient. Structured slab and coil construction can help with sensory integration for adult psychiatric clients (King, 1974).

Psychiatric clients may find it beneficial to make a clay symbol of a person toward whom they feel hostile and then destroy it. Breaking up old dried clay or broken projects of previously discharged clients could be used to achieve a similar goal. In the past, therapists have sometimes felt that wedging or pounding clay helped release aggressive hostility; however for some clients, it may cause the aggression to go to a higher level. The therapist must be very vigilant when using clay with hostile clients, as many clay tools can also become weapons.

Pediatrics

Clay is a natural medium for children. They play in their food, squeezing and manipulating it, in the same way they handle clay. They make mud pies. Clay allows this same kind of unstructured exploration of materials. Many theorists have associated clay with the anal phase in Freud's psychosexual stages, as its texture, color, and consistency resemble feces (Early, 1993).

Children's competency in drawing will be reflected in how they manipulate clay and clay tools. Those who have had little experience in working with art materials or tools usually will not work as long or as independently with clay. They will often produce an unrecognizable lump and move on to more familiar activities. As children show more maturity, they will often name the lump even though it may still be unrecognizable. Gradually, children will begin to make a head, which is separate from the body, and add facial features, progressing in the same developmental way they do in drawing. Pre-adolescent children try to make realistic objects. Younger children may be less intentional about making a permanent object. They are usually more willing to put their clay back into the container after they have satisfied their curiosity and creative urge. Older children and adolescents more often feel strongly about having their objects fired and eventually glazed. While even young children may want the piece fired, they may not care about glazing it (Gaitskell, Hurwitz, 1975). Clay is a common ingredient in play therapy situations. It fits well with the permissiveness of this kind of pediatric treatment. It allows for smearing and the messiness associated with clay and children (Axline, 1947).

Children who have never been allowed to be messy or who have been punished for getting dirty or soiling themselves may have difficulty initially. Eventually most children are able to overcome this sort of anxiety and experience the pure sensual joy of wet clay. The main precautions with this population are ingestion of the materials, and while clay is usually not toxic, glazes are very dangerous and best avoided with small children unless closely supervised. Children tend to make small objects with many appendages such as legs for animals. They almost always break off either before or during firing but can be glued together after firing. If the child has used a mainly two-dimensional scheme, the fired clay can be glued to paper and painted rather than glazed. Many therapists allow children to paint their bisque-fired clay objects with tempera paints rather than glazes. The washability of clay materials also make them a good choice for pediatric bedside therapy.

Geriatrics

Many of the same indicators for therapeutic use of ceramics in physical dysfunction apply to the elderly. In using clay with elderly people, it is best to start out with simple hand-built projects rather than molds, as it is hard to wean them away from molds once they have started. Molds place fewer requirements for creativity and experimentation. However, slip-molded greenware may be a way to entice a regressed elder to begin to participate again in activities. They need to be reminded that the process of making something is more important than a beautiful final product (Weisberg, Wilder, 1985). Because so many elderly people have joint limitations, it is important to help them compensate for this by positioning their projects closer to their bodies.

Elderly people often have sensory loss, such as vision, hearing, and tactile perception. Clay for the visually impaired may provide a creative experience they could not have with something more exacting like needlework. Hearing-impaired clients may be unaware of disturbing another client when wedging, as they cannot hear the noise they are making. People with tactile deficits are in danger of injuring themselves and remaining unaware of the injury. Clay can be incorporated into a memory group by asking, "What does this remind you of?" Such a question will elicit a variety of responses from elders.

CASE STUDY

A 26-year-old married caucasian female, Jean, was admitted to a 20-bed inpatient psychiatric unit in a small private community hospital. Her diagnosis was major depression. Jean and her husband had recently moved to the city from a smaller city where her family lived. She had left her elementary teaching job to follow her engineer husband, whose company had transferred him to a nearby plant. Her symptoms were loss of appetite; weight loss; early morning awakening; complaints of sleepless-

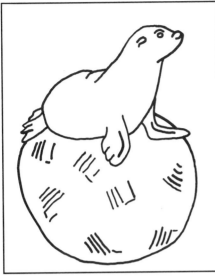

Figure 12-19.
Seal on a rock.

ness, fatigue, decreased attention span, delusional thinking related to contamination of canned and frozen foods; agoraphobia; and suicidal thoughts without concrete plan for accomplishment. The occupational therapist considered herself an eclectic therapist, relying on whichever theory fit the client. She used the Comprehensive Occupational Therapy Evaluation scale because she considered it efficient in showing the greatest amount of information for the amount of time and materials they had. She included the client in a tissue paper flower-making group and observed her during this session. Jean showed mild to moderate dysfunction in all areas except appearance and reality orientation, which were normal. The therapist set goals to increase Jean's activity level as well as self-esteem through continued craft group involvement. At this time, she lacked the insight necessary to participate in her own treatment planning.

The second day, Jean and one other client were the only ones attending the occupational therapy craft group. The therapist presented a variety of craft options to the clients. Jean was unable to make a choice, so the therapist gave her a grapefruit-sized ball of gray clay. She at first seemed unable to decide how to start forming the clay, though she mentioned having used clay with her elementary school students. After several self-deprecatory statements about her inability to do anything good, she began to stroke the clay and manipulate it. By the end of the 1 1/2-hour occupational therapy craft session, she had formed a seal on a rock (Figure 12-19). The therapist helped her cover it with plastic so it would not dry out and could be worked with the next day. At the next session, she used a wire loop tool to hollow out the rock and give it some facets. Two days later, on Friday, it was dry enough to fire along with the projects of several other clients. The client had worked on more paper flowers to decorate her new home on those intervening days.

Over the weekend the kiln cooled down, and on Monday, the client appeared to be lying in wait for the therapist to open the kiln. The nursing staff reported that her medication had been working. She was much more animated. The therapist had warned her as she opened the kiln of the possibility that her seal might have exploded in the kiln because of the thickness of its body. Fortunately, the piece fired well. Jean smiled excitedly when she saw her white bisque-fired seal. She immediately began to select glazes. She chose a glossy black for the seal and a matte green for the rock. That day her physician, with the treatment team, decided she was well enough and stabilized on her medication enough to be discharged. After she packed, she came to the occupational therapist and asked how she would be able to get her seal. The occupational therapist told her she could come by on Thursday to pick it up, as she would be firing the kiln again on Wednesday. When she came to pick it up, she was dressed for a teaching job interview. Jean sat down with the occupational therapist and discussed why she had made the seal. She said she felt like she was stuck out on the rock all alone away from her family and long-time friends. She said she felt that now she was able to get down off the rock and begin to swim again.

The job interview was symbolic of her willingness to face life again. She thanked the therapist and said she'd like to visit again, but she never did. Later the occupational therapist heard from the psychiatrist that Jean had taken a job in a suburban school and was doing well.

DISCUSSION QUESTIONS

1. Would you have done anything differently with Jean? If so, what?
2. What categories of clients might be bothered by the dust from cleaning a seam with a sgraffito tool on a slip-molded object?
3. Do males or females identify more with ceramics? How might this affect their participation? What could you do to get someone to participate who thought clay was something done by the opposite sex?
4. Teenage girls often pay a great deal of attention to beautifying themselves. How could ceramics be used to take advantage of this natural developmental focus?
5. If you used the following questions with clients, what answers might you get when talking with them about their ceramic projects?
   - Were you surprised at the results?
   - Were you able to let go and really work with the clay?
   - What have you learned about yourself?
   - Does this have any bearing on how you handle everyday problems?
6. If the therapist were asked to select one theory model to use with Jean, which of the models in Chapter 2 do you think would be most helpful and why?

REFERENCES

Anonymous. (1986). Hazards in arts & crafts. *Emergency medicine*, 18(18) 60-81.

Axline. V. (1947). *Play therapy*. New York: Ballantine Books.

Budworth, D. W. (1970). *An introduction to ceramic science*. New York: Pergamon Press.

Department of the Army. (1971). *Craft techniques in occupational therapy*. Washington DC: U.S. Government Printing Office.

Dierks, L. (1994). *Creative clay jewelry: Designs to make from polymer clay*. Ashville, NC: Lark Books.

Early, M. B. (1993). *Mental health concepts and techniques for the occupational therapy assistant* (2nd ed.). New York: Raven Press.

Gaitskell, C. D., & Hurwitz, A. (1975). *Children and their art* (3rd ed.). New York: Harcourt, Brace, Jovanovitch.

Hamill, C. M., & Oliver, R. C. (1989). *Therapeutic activity for the handicapped elderly.* Gaithersburg, MD: Aspen Publishers.

Hamilton, D. (1974). *The Thames and Hudson manual of pottery and ceramics.* London: Thames and Hudson Ltd.

Harris, D. B. (1963). *Children's drawings as measures of intellectual maturity.* New York: Harcourt, Brace and World, Inc.

Hemphill, B. J. (1982). *The evaluative process in psychiatric occupational therapy.* Thorofare, NJ: SLACK Incorporated.

King, L. J. (1974). A sensory integrative approach to schizophrenia. *Am J Occup Ther, 28*(9), 529-536.

Marmer, L. (1997). Ceramics for business and pleasure: Why John Q. Public is embracing an art of antiquity. *Advance for Occupational Therapists, 13*(28), 14-15.

Moyer, B. (1983). *Index of assessments used by occupational therapists in mental health.* Monograph. Rockville, MD: American Occupational Therapy Association.

Nelson, G. C. (1966) *Ceramics: A potter's handbook* (2nd ed.). New York: Holt, Rinehart and Winston.

O'Kane, C. P. (1968). *The development of a projective technique for use in psychiatric occupational therapy.* Buffalo: State University of New York.

Turoff, M. P. (1949). *How to mMake pottery and other ceramic ware.* New York: Crown Publishers.

Weisberg, N., & Wilder, R. (1985). *Creative arts with older adults: A sourcebook.* New York: Human Sciences Press.

Wettlaufer, G., & Wettlaufer, N. (1976). *Getting into pots: A basic pottery manual.* Englewood Cliffs, NJ: Prentice Hall.

Wilkinson, V. C., & Heater, S. L. (1979). *Therapeutic media and techniques of application: A guide for activities therapists.* New York: Van Nostrand Reinhold Company.

WEAVING, LATCHHOOK, MACRAMÉ & OTHER FIBER CRAFTS

INTRODUCTION

Fiber crafts include much more than those mentioned in this chapter. To include all fiber crafts is out of the realm of this text. The most commonly used crafts for occupational therapy will be discussed, with only two examples being described in detail.

FIBER CRAFTS USED IN OCCUPATIONAL THERAPY

Weaving

After leather, wood, and ceramics, weaving may be the next craft that humans developed. It probably grew out of a tradition of basketry, which is also weaving. Grasses, reeds, and leaves were probably the first woven fibers. Because of their vegetable nature, few of these early weaving artifacts have survived. The Middle Eastern cultures documented their crafts in artwork, such as murals, as well as commercial records like clay tablets. We know that cloth was being woven in 4500 BC, however, almost all indigenous cultures have developed a form of weaving or basketry (Department of the Army, 1971; Moseley, Johnson, Koenig, 1962; *Reader's Digest*, 1979).

Weaving can be as simple as paper weaving, which is dealt with in the next chapter, or it can be as complex as that done on a four-harness floor

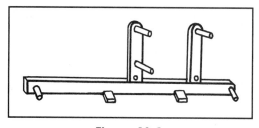

Figure 13-1.
Inkle loom.

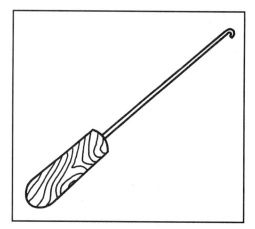

Figure 13-2.
Rug hook.

loom. Basically, no matter what the fiber, it is the same process—interweaving one set of strands with another set at right angles. The longitudinal threads are called the warp, while the latitudinal strands are termed weft or woof (Hedrick, 1971; Scharff, 1952).

In the past in occupational therapy clinics, it was common to see looms in use. There were often adapted looms to be used over a bed or positioned to require clients to use shoulder flexion, adduction, and abduction (Department of the Army, 1971; Colson, 1944; Haworth, MacDonald, 1946; Willard, Spackman, 1947). It is possible for many looms to be "homemade"(Moseley, Johnson, Koenig, 1962; Alexander, 1969; Harding, 1973). Some kinds of weaving require little equipment, such as the inkle loom (Figure 13-1), finger weaving, card weaving, and stick weaving. All of these are forms of strip weaving. The strips are then used as bracelets, belts, headbands, and hat bands, or are sewn together to make rugs or blankets. Knitting and crocheting are forms of making fabric without having threads interwoven at right angles. God's Eyes, which are a traditional Mexican and Indian decorative craft, are another kind of weaving that most beginners can do successfully (Stribling, 1973).

Latchhook

Latchhook is a modern adaptation of a common older style of rug-making called knotting or Turkish knotting, which can be made on any flat loom. It is a way of knotting fringe through two warp threads at a time. Row after row of fringe produces a nice pile rug (Department of the Army, 1971; Moseley, Johnson, Koenig, 1962). Hooked rugs were often made with a burlap backing. A rug hook, which is a simple hook set in a wooden handle (Figure 13-2), is used to pull loops of yarn up through the burlap to make a pile (*Better Homes and Gardens*, 1966).

Carpets today are essentially made in the same way, though done by machine. Some have cut pile, which is like Turkish knotting, and some have looped piles like hooked rugs (Department of the Army, 1971;

Scharff, 1952). A latchhook is a special kind of hook with a small hinged appendage on it, which helps automatically knot the yarn as it is pulled through the rug canvas. The canvas is heavy woven, white, coarse cloth with large holes for inserting the latchhook. It can be purchased in kits or rolls and cut to size. The yarn pieces used in latchooking are 2 to 4 inches in length. They can be purchased ready-cut or can be cut on a special yarn cutter that cuts it directly from the skein. Latchhook projects often take more time than is available in today's short-stay hospitals. However, once the process of latching is learned, it is an easy repetitive task. Latchhook projects can be used for pillows, toilet covers, chair pads, and rugs. Perhaps the most difficult part of latchooking is finishing the edges, as the canvas is stiff and scratchy. Consequently it is difficult to fold over and stitch.

Macramé

This ancient craft of knotting was used by the pharonic Egyptians, Chinese, Maoris, and Peruvians. The word *macramé* has an Arabic origin meaning a veil of protection or a towel or napkin with a fringe. Because many of the knots used in macramé were also used by sailors, it is probable that the skill migrated to new places via the sea (Moseley, Johnson, Koenig, 1962; *Reader's Digest,* 1979).

Macramé can be accomplished with almost no tools. Some therapists use special macramé boards and pins, but this is not necessary. Many macramé projects are time consuming and consequently not appropriate for a short hospital stay. Simple projects can be done with tools already on hand in the clinic, such as scissors and masking tape.

In simple macramé, there are four basic knots with several variations for each (Octopus Books, 1973). There are more than 30 complicated knots that can be incorporated if the activity needs to be graded up (Abraham, 1964). This craft can easily be graded up or down, and the range of projects may include key chains, belts, purses, shopping bags, jewelry, wall hangings, and plant pot hangers (*Reader's Digest,* 1979).

FREQUENCY OF USE

Between 5% and 20% of therapists use macramé as often as one time per week or more. Many others use macramé occasionally or less than once a week (Titus, 1997).

In working on specific occupational therapy goals, weaving and latchhook are often used to improve group socialization. Turkish knotting and knitting are used to increase bilateral dexterity. Latchhook weaving and macramé are used to improve fine motor control. Some therapists use weaving to provide an outlet for frustration.

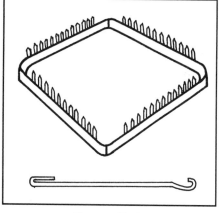

Figure 13-3.
Looper frame and hook.

ASSESSMENTS

Informal assessment of cognition, perceptual–motor, visual–perceptual, and fine motor functions are possible using fiber crafts. Formal assessments usually do not use fibers. Perhaps this is because fiber crafts are an entirely new, complicated process to many clients. Such an evaluation, which would involve teaching the craft, would test only a narrow range of learning skills such as memory, following instructions, etc. The Neuropsychiatric Interest (NPI) checklist includes knitting on its list of 80 activities. No other fiber arts except sewing and embroidery, which are classified in this text as needlework, are included. On the NPI checklist, the client marks casual, strong, or none to indicate the level of interest in each activity (Matsutsuya, 1969).

Making Loopers

Loopers are simple squares woven from cotton or nylon jersey loops. Aside from paper weaving, they are the simplest weaving project. Perhaps that is why they are so commonly used.

SUPPLIES

- Looper frame (Figure 13-3)
- Color assortment of loopers
- Wire looper hook

PROCESS

Each side of the looper frame has 18 prongs:
1. Number each side of the frame.
2. Start on side one and slip a looper over the first prong, pull it across and hook it on the first prong directly across on side three.
3. Continue until loopers are hooked around the opposite prong on sides one and three. This is the warp.
4. To interweave the weft, starting on side two, slide the wire looper hook through the warp going under, over, under, over.
5. Slip the hook through the looper. Then slide the looper over the first prong on side two and pull the looper through the warp. Hook it on the side four prong opposite the one where it is hooked on side two.

Some consider each looper as one strand. It is perhaps less confusing for beginners to go under, over, under, over, considering each side of one looper as a separate strand. Either way is satisfactory, though the two-strand method gives a more vivid contrast of the colors. This plain weave is called "tabby." Contrasting colors can be used to make a plaid effect. When each of the 18 weft loopers is woven through the warp and attached to the prongs at both sides, the square is ready to be removed.

6. Start at the same corner where the first warp looper was hooked over the prong on side one. Gently lift the next loop off the next prong.

7. Pull the second loop through the first. The hook will remain in the second loop, ready to lift off the third loop, and pull it through the second.

8. Continue until all loops are pulled through the previous loop. It may be necessary to pull a strand on the finished edge over a prong on each side to keep the square in place until the last loop is taken off the prong.

9. The finishing touch is to take another looper and put it through the last loop to make a hanger if the square is to be used as a potholder.

10. These squares can also be sewn together for rugs and placemats (Alexander, 1969).

Macramé Key Chain

Making macramé key chains is a simple project that can often be finished in one session to satisfy clients who need immediate gratification. The simplest key chain uses just two strands of cord. Macramé can be graded up from more strands on the key chain to complex wall hangings or clothing.

SUPPLIES

- One split key ring
- Two spools of different colored macramé cord
- Assorted beads
- Yardstick
- Scissors
- Masking tape

PROCESS

1. Tape the key ring to the table approximately 12 inches from the edge at the place where the client will sit.

2. Cut 1 yard of each color of cord.

3. Dip the ends of the cord in lacquer or nail polish so they won't fray during the macramé process. Allow these to dry. This is not always necessary, but some clients tend to cause the cords to fray from

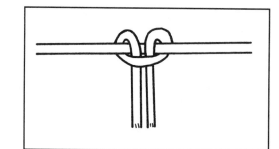

Figure 13-4.
Larkshead knot.

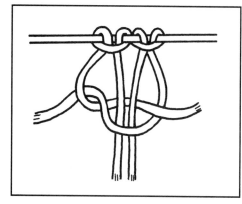

Figure 13-5.
Square knot starting with the right.

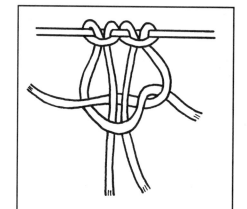

Figure 13-6.
Square knot starting with the left.

too much handling. If the client doesn't want to put beads on the macramé, the ends can be separately knotted in overhand knots to keep the ends from fraying.

4. Fold the cords in half and knot each strand through the key ring using a larkshead knot (Figure 13-4).
5. Tape the two center holding cords down to the table.
6. Lay the right-hand cord across the two holding cords and place the left under the holding cords; pull it over the right cord and through the loop (Figure 13-5).
7. Next lay the left cord across the two holding cords. Place the right end over the end of the left cord, under the holding cords and up through the loop (Figure 13-6).
8. Continue in this way.
9. After several knots, the client may desire to put a bead on the two holding strands.
10. At this point, the two outer strands can be taped down and become the holding strands. Then the previous holding strands, which are

longer at this point, are the ones used to make the knots as described above.

11. When the macramé reaches the desired length, cut off the extra cord.

12. The client may want to put a bead near the end of each of the four strands and tie an overhand knot at the bottom to keep the beads from sliding off.

MAIN THERAPEUTIC APPLICATIONS

Physical Dysfunction

Floor looms were once considered the most adaptable piece of craft equipment for working on range of motion, strength, and endurance of both lower and upper extremities. They are seldom found in rehabilitation clinics today, possibly because of their floorspace requirements. Clients with ataxia or cerebellar dysfunction can practice movements in weaving that are normally controlled by the cerebellum, such as starting, stopping, and balance. Practice can allow the client to learn to control these movements cortically. Those with hemiparesis can practice bilateral hand activity in all of the activities discussed in this chapter. The blind and deaf receive much tactile input through weaving and macramé. The small projects described in this chapter are easy to use in bed for confined clients. If clients have allergies or respiratory problems, caution needs to be used in choosing lint-free cord and yarn.

Mental Health

The simple fiber arts are appropriate for clients with poor attention spans. These activities are highly structured for clients who are, for example, schizophrenic and manic. These crafts offer quick gratification. They include simple skills that, once learned, can easily be built upon. Depressed clients who tire easily usually have enough endurance for these kinds of small projects. Latchhook may seem a little more difficult to learn and certainly takes longer to complete. One precaution with fiber crafts is that suicidal clients may be tempted to try to hang themselves with cord. It is best not to let them take such projects to their rooms. The educable mentally retarded (IQ 50–70) who can achieve academic skills to the 6th grade can benefit from structured activities such as crochet, simple weaving, latchhook, and simple macramé. The repetitive nature of these crafts is non-threatening to the mentally retarded (APA, 1994).

Pediatrics

Fiber crafts are too difficult for most young children. Older children enjoy simple fiber crafts. Boys may be motivated to try macramé, as it will prepare them to learn nautical skills. Both boys and girls can enjoy weaving. If a boy suggests that it is not masculine, the therapist can describe how men do the weaving in countries like Saudi Arabia. Children may find latchhook an especially satisfying activity if they work on the rug canvas with large holes using the very thickest yarn to make the pile plush enough. Simple patterns lend themselves to thick yarn (MacFarlan, 1973). There are many informal materials that can be used in children's weavings, such as dead tree branches, large pieces of bark, cardboard, and twine (Carlson, 1993).

Geriatrics

Fiber activities are often chosen by older women. Many of them have had crotchet hooks or knitting needles in their hands since childhood. In these cases, fiber activities need little teaching. For older people, it is often best to let them do what they know well, as success in these activities can do much for failing self-esteem. Many men have learned to tie a variety of knots in their work or in home maintenance. This skill makes macramé a natural activity for them as well. They can craft gifts for friends or family.

Fiber crafts are inexpensive compared to wood, leather, and ceramics, which makes them attractive activities for use in nursing homes and other long-term care facilities that have limited craft budgets.

Fiber crafts are not breakable. This is an important feature for geriatric clients who, because of their balance problems, may drop things (Gould, Gould, 1971).

CASE STUDY

Helen is a 21-year-old caucasian female who is classified as moderately mentally retarded with an IQ of 50. She lives with her parents in a suburban neighborhood. She is their only child remaining at home. For the past 12 years she has ridden a bus for special education students across town to a school that has classes for the retarded. She also has epilepsy, which is controlled by medication. For the past 7 years, the school's occupational therapist, who uses Developmental/Spatiotemporal Adaptation Theory, has been working with Helen's teacher to develop her work skills in preparation for future placement in a sheltered workshop. At age 14, they started her on a program of standing for 15 minutes to do a repetitive task, gradually increasing her standing tolerance by 5-minute increments. Some of the activities she did during this training were sorting colored objects, stringing beaded necklaces as gifts, making a link belt, using scissors to cut out coupons, and cooking simple dishes. They were felt to be positive experiences for her developmental level as well as her age.

By the time she was 21 years old, she had a standing tolerance of 2 hours. At this age, she was no longer eligible for special education services, so the occupational therapist worked with other school personnel to help Helen make a smooth transition to the sheltered workshop. She accompanied Helen on a visit to the workshop. The workshop had a full-time certified occupational therapy assistant (COTA) and a contract occupational therapist who spent 4 hours per week evaluating clients. The two occupational therapists set up a telephone conference concerning Helen. During her first 2 weeks at the workshop, she began to have seizures again. A call to her parents verified that she had been taking her medication. The workshop required that she start wearing her protective helmet again. Because her seizures had been controlled for so many years, she had not been made to wear it. The pediatrician whom Helen had been seeing for years consented to see her again, though he had been trying to get her referred to a family practice clinic that served many mentally retarded clients. The pediatrician began to alter her medication in an attempt to control the seizures.

The occupational therapist in the sheltered workshop evaluated Helen at the end of the second week and found her to be unkempt, sluggish, and unresponsive. She got up and began to wander around the occupational therapy room during the evaluation. She started to go through the occupational therapist's desk saying, "Candy! Candy!" Her behavior did not fit with the description given by the school therapist. The workshop occupational therapist decided to call the school to discuss this situation. The outcome was to try to reduce Helen's stress level by allowing her a more gradual integration into the workshop program. Usually, the workshop van brought the clients at 8:30 a.m. At 9 a.m., they started on the day's work. At the end of each hour there was a 10-minute break. At 11:00 a.m., the COTA taught a trainable mentally retarded vocational class. Helen was enrolled in this class. From 11:45 a.m. to 12:30 p.m., clients ate their lunch in the workshop cafeteria. At 12:30 p.m. they returned to work for 2 hours. From 2:30 until 3:30 p.m., the COTA had a craft group for those clients who had been on time, dressed neatly, and who had worked well.

The occupational therapist and COTA made the following goals, and Helen agreed to work on these goals:
- To be punctual at her work station
- To be neatly dressed and groomed
- To stay at her work station for 50 minutes
- To finish one task before starting another
- To perform age appropriate work 5 hours per day

It was decided that the COTA would work on some of these skills in the TMR vocational class and decide on Helen's rewards in the craft session. Helen had initially indicated interest in several crafts. She had never done looper weaving. At the next session, the COTA had Helen sort out loopers for weaving into four separate colors and put each color in a separate bag. The next day she allowed Helen to choose the two colors she would like to use in her own looper. She chose blue and green. Though the COTA felt they did not look good together, she did not interfere because she felt Helen needed more independent decision making. At that session, Helen put the blue warp loopers on the loom. The following day, Helen completed weaving the green weft loopers. On the third day, she had difficulty with the process of removing the loops from the prongs and hooking them through the previous loop. The COTA had to sit beside her to see that she was doing it correctly. Finally, after she reached the fourth side of the loom, she seemed to catch on to this process. She was proud of the completed potholder and took it to show each person in the clinic saying, "Isn't it pretty?"

She told the COTA she wanted to make another one. The COTA said if she came to her work station on time and was neat and clean she could start another the next day. Helen responded positively to this agreement. Her seizures began to diminish and eventually disappeared. It was felt by the workshop staff that the simple repetitive nature of looper weaving seemed to calm Helen and reduce her stress, which was believed to have set off the seizures. While Helen did later learn other crafts, nothing seemed to please her like loopers.

DISCUSSION QUESTIONS

1. What particular features of loopers might appeal so strongly to Helen?
2. How could the COTA grade up loopers to keep a higher-functioning client interested and challenged?
3. Which of the fiber crafts described in this chapter requires the greatest range of motion?

REFERENCES

Abraham, R. M. (1964). *Diversions and pastimes with coins, cards, string, paper and matches.* New York; Dover Publications.

Alexander, M. (1969). *Simple weaving.* New York: Tower Publications.

American Psychiatric Association. (1994). *Diagnostic and statistical manual of mental disorders, DSM-IV* (4th ed.). Washington DC: American Psychiatric Association.

Better Homes and Gardens. (1966). *Stitchery and crafts.* New York: Meredith Press.

Carlson, L. (1993) *EcoArt: Earth friendly art & craft experiences for 3-to 9-year-olds.* Charlotte, VT: Williamson Publishing.

Colson, J. H. C. (1944). *The rehabilitation of the injured: Occupational therapy.* London: Cassell and Company.

Department of the Army. (1971). *Craft techniques in occupational therapy.* Washington DC: U.S. Government Printing Office

Gould, E. & Gould, L. (1971). *Crafts for the elderly.* Springfield, IL: Charles C. Thomas Publishers.

Harding, D. (February 1973). Weaving with a simple stick loom. *Family Circle, 81,* 152,154.

Haworth, N. A., & MacDonald, E. M. (1946). *Theory of occupational therapy.* Baltimore: Williams & Wilkins.

Hedrick, S. J. (Ed.). (1971). *What shall I weave?* Shelby, NC: Lily Mills Company.

MacFarlan, A.S. (1973). T*he boys book of rainy-day-doings.* New York: Galahad Books.

Matsutsuya, J. S. (1969). The interest checklist. *Am J Occup Ther, 24*(4), 323-328.

Moseley, S., Johnson, P,. & Koenig, H. (1962). *Crafts design.* Belmont, CA: Wadsworth.

Octopus Books. (1973). *The basic book of macramé and tatting.* Hong Kong: Mandarin Publishers.

Reader's Digest. (1979). *Crafts and hobbies.* Pleasantville, NY: Reader's Digest Association, Inc.

Scharff, R. (1952). *Handbook of crafts.* Greenville, CT: Fawcett Publications.

Stribling, M. L. (1973). *Art from found materials.* New York: Crown Publishers, Inc.

Titus, J. (1997). Treatment interventions used on level II occupational therapy fieldwork. Unpublished manuscript.

Willard, H. S., & Spackman. C. S. (1947). *Principles of occupational therapy.* Philadelphia: Lippincott.

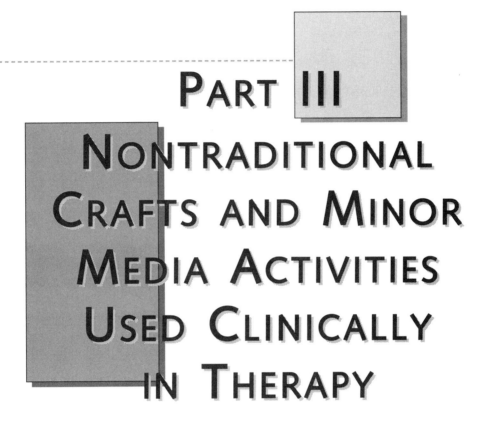

PART III

NONTRADITIONAL CRAFTS AND MINOR MEDIA ACTIVITIES USED CLINICALLY IN THERAPY

PAPER CRAFTS

INTRODUCTION

Paper was invented in China sometime between 200 and 100 B.C. Other materials had been used to write on for many centuries before that: wet clay, tree bark, cloth, and papyrus, from which the word paper comes. Early paper was used almost solely to write on. The Arabs who learned about paper from their conquests in Asia introduced it to Europe.

Paper was still being made by hand at the time of the invention of the printing press in the 15th century. In the 18th century, a machine was invented that could make paper from wood pulp, though it did not become widely used for another 100 years. During this time, the Chinese had been developing glue they used to fashion many paper crafts. The Chinese continue to make cut paper ornaments from recycled paper even today. The Japanese craft of paper folding, origami, became increasingly sophisticated, and today there is a tradition of groups joining in folding 1,000 paper cranes as expressions of peace and love. Mexican paper cutouts are intricate and colorful. The French developed the craft of papier mâché or chewed paper.

Paper is perhaps our cheapest and most available craft material. Almost every office has a supply of paper, pencils, glue, scissors, tape, staples, and paper clips—all that are needed for many projects. Most of us have been doing paper crafts for so long we seldom think of them as important, but they can be adapted for almost any client population. Our parents may have kept us quiet at church, mosque, or temple by folding paper boats. We learned how to outwit our teachers by flying paper airplanes. Our earliest party and holiday decorations may have been paper chains. Paper, aside from its important function for writing, offers a world of craft delight for all ages (Department of the Army, 1971; Moseley, Johnson, Koenig, 1962; *Reader's Digest*, 1979).

A recent popular craft activity/occupation is paper making, or sometimes called paper casting. This involves making a pulp from soft tissue or using ready-prepared fibers. The pulp is then pressed into a terra cotta clay mold and allowed to dry. These castings can be painted, glued, and punched to make decorations (Barron, 1992).

FREQUENCY OF USE

Collage, decoupage, and nature printing are among the most commonly used paper crafts (Titus, 1997). Only one of these, collage, will be discussed in this chapter. The paper crafts described here are mostly three-dimensional crafts or at least those involving folding the paper before cutting it. While folded paper crafts may be less commonly used than other crafts such as woodworking, they have the remarkable potential to increase visual motor integration, spatial operations, fine coordination/dexterity, motor control, sequencing, and other cognitive processes such as memory. The low cost of this treatment material is another reason why therapists use it more frequently.

ASSESSMENTS

Perhaps because paper crafts do not seem sophisticated to therapists, or therapists think clients may consider such activities as beneath them in relation to their age, few formal assessments include paper crafts. The Fidler Activity Laboratory includes two paper activities (Hemphill, 1982). The first is a drawing of a chicken, which the client is asked to cut out and reproduce on another sheet of paper. The second is a collage using a variety of colored paper, objects, and glue. The first offers almost no opportunity for creativity, but the second activity can be quite imaginative. Other activities in this battery include fingerpainting and negotiating an obstacle course.

The Build-a-City assessment is a projective test meant primarily for testing a group of children. The assessment's author, however, lists the age span for the assessment from toddler to geriatric. This assessment does work especially well with children. Colored construction paper, along with tape, string, clay, pipe cleaners, scissors, and clay tools are provided. The therapist simply asks the group of 5 to 8 clients to build an ideal city. Interaction, fine coordination/dexterity, other motor performance skills, and the approach to the task can be assessed (AOTA Practice Division, 1988).

The Lafayette Clinic Battery for children 6 to 10 years of age uses construction paper, scissors, pencils, paste, and circle patterns to test eye-hand coordination (Llorens, 1969). The test also includes a geometric form worksheet and puzzle. This assessment evaluates the child's developmental skills.

The Magazine Picture Collage is an adult psychiatric occupational therapy evaluation. In this assessment, the client is given colored construction paper, a pile of magazines, scissors, and glue. The client is asked to look for pictures that appeal to him or her and glue them to the construction paper. This assessment has been well validated for interrater reliability (Hemphill, 1982).

Papier Mâché

Papier mâché can be made by several different processes: by soaking pieces of torn up newspaper and mixing it with cooked starch; by using commercially prepared papier mâché mix; or by using the strip method. The last method will be discussed here, as illustrated by the creation of a papier mâché wall mask.

SUPPLIES
- Paper plate
- Newspapers
- Masking tape
- Liquid white glue
- Bowl to mix glue
- Tempera paints and brushes

PROCESS
1. Cover the work space with several layers of newspaper.
2. Make a mask form by loosely wadding several pieces of newspaper and taping them into the top of the paper plate to make the general shape of a face.
3. If a nose or other appendage such as ears or beard are desired, small wads of paper can be taped on the form.
4. Cover as much of the surface with tape as possible, as it will allow the finished mask to be more easily removed from the plate and wadded paper.
5. Tear up one sheet of black and white newspaper into strips approximately 1 inch wide.
6. In the bowl, mix one part white glue to one part water.
7. Dip each strip in the glue/water mixture and apply it to the mask form. Allow this to dry thoroughly before applying the next layer of strips. This may take 24 hours.
8. For the next layer, tear strips from the colored comic strip section of the newspaper so that when the glued strips are applied, it is easy to see that all the surface has been covered with the second

layer. Allow this to dry as well. The third and last layer of strips should be of plain black and white newspaper.

9. After the third layer is dry, smooth the mask by lightly sanding the surface or by adding additional strips to rough spots.
10. Pull off the paper plate and wadded paper when the mask is completely dry.
11. Paint the mask with any water-based paint.
12. Lacquer the mask to keep the paint from wearing off.

If the mask is to be worn, rather than hung on the wall, leave eye holes on the very first as well as subsequent layers. It is better not to try to cut the completely dried mask, as it may crack (Moseley, Johnson, Koenig, 1962; Reader's Digest, 1979). Mask-making kits are available that include plaster gauze used for making plaster casts. The uniformity of the masks from the plastic mold appeals to clients who feel unable to construct their own face mold from newspaper. However, there is less creativity used in making a mask on a mold.

Paper Weaving

This craft is appropriate for almost any age. It can help assess and improve clients' awareness of space, awareness of under and over or spacial relations, fine motor coordination, and motor praxis. The process for making a simple woven placemat is described below.

SUPPLIES
- Two 12 x 18-inch sheets of different colored construction paper
- Scissors (be sure to have left-handed scissors available)
- White glue

PROCESS
1. Decide on which color the background, or warp, will be, as described in the chapter on fiber crafts.
2. Fold that sheet lengthwise down the middle.
3. Mark the edge opposite the fold so there is a 1/2-inch margin.
4. Start from the fold and cut to the margin, making cuts 3/4 inch apart (Figure 14-1).
5. Open up the sheet and lay it flat.
6. From the other sheet, cut 3/4-inch lengthwise weft strips (Figure 14-2).
7. To make a plain tabby weave, take one weft strip and go under, over, under, over.
8. The next strip will be over, under, over, under.
9. Continue weaving, alternating these patterns until there is no more room for a weft to be woven into the warp (Figure 14-3).
10. Lightly glue the ends of each weft strip.

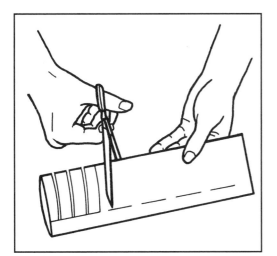

Figure 14-1.
Cutting warp for paper weaving.

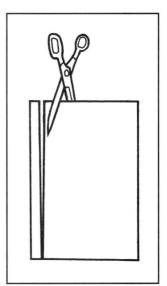

Figure 14-2.
Cutting weft for
paper weaving.

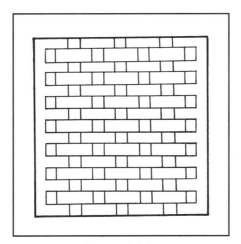

Figure 14-3.
Completed paper weaving.

Folded Paper

The Japanese are famous for their origami figures. Because it is a traditional craft in Japan, almost every Japanese school child learns to create some figures. Animals, flowers, puppets, boxes, and abstract forms are all subjects for the origami crafter. Many of these forms can be adapted for use in the clinic. The cat shown in the following illustrations is one of the simplest figures. It is possible to buy special origami paper, but any thin paper such as typing paper can be used.

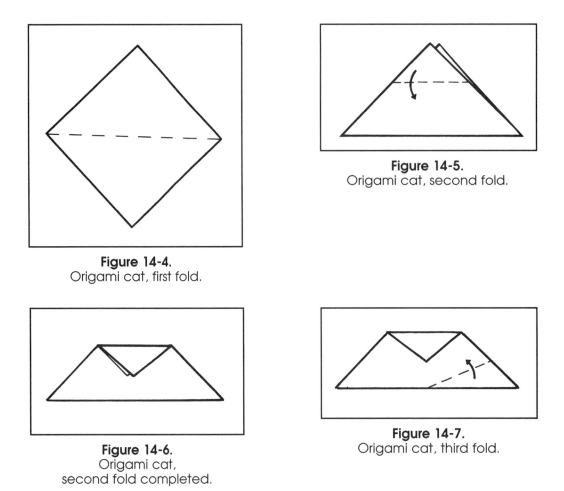

Figure 14-4.
Origami cat, first fold.

Figure 14-5.
Origami cat, second fold.

Figure 14-6.
Origami cat,
second fold completed.

Figure 14-7.
Origami cat, third fold.

PROCESS

1. Fold an 8-inch square of paper from corner to corner (Figure 14-4).
2. Next fold the top corner so the crease comes 2 inches from the top corner (Figures 14-5 and 14-6).
3. Fold the ears up (Figures 14-7, 14-8, and 14-9), and turn the cat's head over.
4. Draw eyes, nose, mouth, and whiskers. The cat's face can be decorated in a number of different ways (Figure 14-10) (Sakade, 1958).

Paper Sculpture

Paper sculpture offers an infinite variety for stimulating creativity. Subjects can be realistic, futuristic, imaginative, or abstract. Glue is the next most important material after paper for this kind of sculpture (Bottomley, 1983; Fabri, 1966). Sculpture implies that it is a three-dimensional object. Sculpture can be constructed from a pattern (Figure 14-11), or it can be built by adding paper to an understructure.

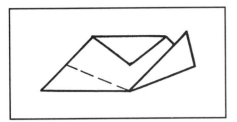

Figure 14-8.
Origami cat, fourth and final fold.

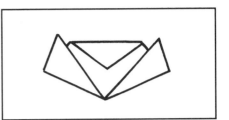

Figure 14-9.
Back of the origami cat face.

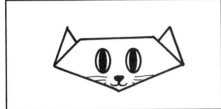

Figure 14-10.
Front of origami cat face
drawn on with felt pen.

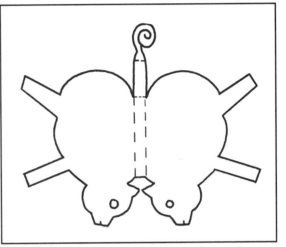

Figure 14-11.
Paper sculpture pattern.

The piñata described in this chapter uses the latter technique. A piñata is a Mexican holiday sculpture used as a game. The outcome of the game is a broken piñata, but it can be appropriate fun in some situations.

SUPPLIES

- Two large brown paper bags
- Cellophane tape
- Large needles and string
- Assorted wrapped candies
- Colored tissue paper
- Glue
- Water
- Scissors

PROCESS

1. Fit one paper bag inside the other.
2. Fold 2 inches of the tops of both bags down inside the bags.
3. Place a strip of cellophane tape on the middle where the string will

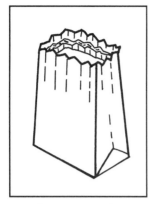

Figure 14-12.
Accordion-folded
bag with taped strip
for piñata.

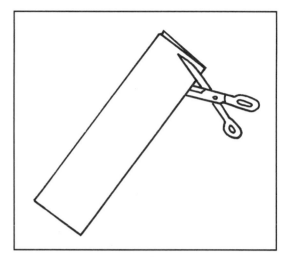

Figure 14-13.
Cut the folded edge of
the tissue paper strip.

go through. That will reinforce the paper so the string won't tear the bags as easily.

4. Now, accordion fold the folded tops of the bags.
5. Put needle and string through this taped strip (Figure 14-12).
6. Fill the double bag with candy to approximately 5 inches from the top.
7. Pull the string to close the top of the bag. Leave the extra string at the top to hang the piñata. Now the piñata structure is ready to be covered with fringed paper. This shape makes a nice piece of fruit, like an apple or a berry.
8. The piñata can be hung up during the gluing process. Take a 4 x 24-inch length of tissue paper and fold it down the middle.
9. Cut 1/4-inch widths (Figure 14-13) along the length of the strip.
10. Glue the uncut edges of the folded paper to the piñata structure starting at the bottom and working in a spiral until the whole piñata is covered. Use the glue sparingly, spreading it with a small brush.
11. Near the string, add a few rows of green fringe to make it look like a fruit stem. Allow the piñata to dry for at least 24 hours.

The piñata game is played by tying a rope to the piñata string so it can be pulled up or let down lower. A basketball hoop makes a good place to hang a piñata, so there is enough space underneath to play the game. All the players form a big circle around the piñata. Each player is blindfolded in turn. They are led to the center of the circle and given one half or one fourth of a turn before they are allowed to try to break the piñata with a stick (Figure 14-14). Care must be taken that all the players in the cir-

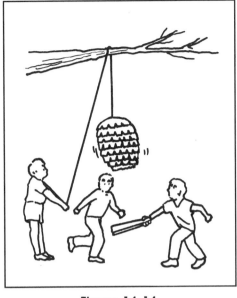

Figure 14-14.
Children breaking the piñata.

cle stay far out of the reach of the stick. Turns are taken hitting at the piñata until someone breaks it and the candy falls on the ground. All players share the candy. This Mexican game is often played at Christmas. It can also be played at any special occasion, such as a client's birthday.

MAIN THERAPEUTIC APPLICATIONS

Physical Dysfunction

Paper crafts can be structured for almost any health care situation. They are especially appropriate for home health clients, as the materials are usually available and not costly to replace. Most of the paper crafts emphasize finger, wrist, forearm, and elbow movement. While little strength is required in most cases, endurance may be required to hold pieces of paper in a position until the glue or starch sticks. Paper crafts are especially good for cardiac and respiratory clients, as little exertion is required. All motion can be done in the lap. The materials give off no toxic fumes. Almost all paper crafts require bilateral hand function and motor control.

Mental Health

Paper craft is potentially frustrating, as paper can readily tear or be crushed. The therapist must be very alert to those clients who need closer supervision to prevent failure. Psychiatric clients often have difficulty judging how much glue to use. Applying the glue with a small brush may help with this problem.

Simple paper folding can be used to assess cognitive function, ability to follow directions, spatial operations, and frustration tolerance. For the higher-functioning client, paper sculpture can be used as a projective test in the same way other sculpture is used. Clients can be asked to describe their sculpture and indicate what meaning it has for them.

Paper crafts make wonderful holiday decorations. Hanging ornaments, flowers, garlands, streamers, and mobiles all help to bring a holiday mood to a clinic or dayroom. Most paper crafts, except paper weaving and paper chains, will be too difficult for mentally retarded clients. However, they may enjoy drawing round stencils, cutting them out, and pasting them onto another color of paper.

Pediatrics

Paper crafts are especially good for children, as they can use their own creations as toys. Very young children can tear paper, but they very quickly want to use scissors. They can make paper puppets or paper bag puppets who do their talking for them, which is especially appropriate for children having difficulty communicating. They can build a world, destroy it, and rebuild it, as they do in their fantasies. They can make their own family members or pets and do to them whatever they fantasize, as an emotional release.

One of the greatest problems for children is that they use too much glue. Paste may be better for young children, though it does not hold as well. Cone-based structures are best for paper sculpture, as they usually create no balance problems. Children are particularly likely to form sculptures with a base too small to support them. Children often want to embellish their paper craft with paint or crayon. Encouragement of such creativity will foster more exploration of materials and possibilities. As children approach adolescence, they want to make more realistic sculptures. Paper craft does not lend itself to realism in most situations. Drawing may be better for this age. However, teens can excel at mask making, origami, and sculpture (Gaitskell, Hurwitz, 1975; Hainsworth, Siqueland, 1969).

Geriatrics

Paper and fabric can often be used to make similar designs. Quilt patterns and applique that may have been used by the clients in the past can easily be adapted to paper designs. Few older clients like to experiment, so the kinds of projects they will enjoy are often fairly familiarly structured activities. Even the most disabled clients in nursing homes often enjoy pasting precut flowers into a bouquet or precut holly leaves into a wreath. This offers opportunities for ensured success. Making paper toys for children may provide stimulation for some elderly clients. Paper crafts may be difficult for a client with vision problems. Folding paper could stress severely deformed arthritic finger and hand joints. Paper cuts from the edge of the paper are painful and annoying. Particular precautions need to be taken with the elderly clients who heal more slowly.

CASE STUDY

In a children's mental health unit with a bed capacity of 10, the occupational therapist performed almost all client evaluation and treatment in a group setting. Most of the clients had the diagnosis of conduct disorder, though occasionally there were others. The programs had strict behavioral limits. Children earned privileges such as television or playground time through accomplishing goals for each treatment session, mealtime, and therapeutic community meeting. The theories most frequently used in this clinic were neuromotor behavior and learning/cognitive disabilities.

There was an adolescent treatment unit next door. Clients were placed in whichever program they best fit behaviorally. The average length of stay was 3 weeks. The occupational therapist split her time between these two psychiatric units. On the children's unit, she customarily evaluated each child individually with the Meeting Street School Screening Test to assess information processing capabilities and gross and fine motor development (Hainsworth, Siqueland, 1969). The Draw-A-Person test was administered in a group if possible, as was the Build-a-City assessment.

Since programming was slightly less structured on weekends and children were often discharged before weekends, the evaluation was usually done by Friday to ensure enough children for a group. A certified occupational therapy assistant (COTA) came in for 4 hours each weekend day to do the occupational therapy treatment programs.

Seven-year-old Ronald was admitted on a Friday, which was an unusual occurrence. The hospital usually tried not to make admissions on Friday, so new clients would not come into the less-structured weekend program. However, Ronald's single mother said she could not care for him another minute. She had three younger children living with her in her mother's house. Her mother was unable to help her with childcare, as she is physically disabled. Ronald had been attacking his younger siblings and endangering himself by jumping off high places and riding his bike off cement culverts. He was just recovering from a broke arm. The psychiatrist diagnosed Ronald as suffering from depression with conduct disorder.

The occupational therapist administered the Meeting Street School Screening Test and found Ronald performed normally on gross and fine motor tasks, though his responses were sometimes slightly delayed. There was some interference in his information processing. Though he performed tasks adequately, he seemed inattentive. His projective story about the two figures involved stealing a cat and hurting it.

The therapist had to postpone the other two tests. She discussed Ronald's condition by telephone with the weekend COTA. On Monday morning, Tom and Paul, two brothers ages 6 and 8 years, were admitted. They had been taken from their foster home and brought to the hospital by the case worker. The psychiatrist in the psychiatric daycare had seen them both before, but this was their first hospital admission. They were both diagnosed with conduct disorders.

Their mother had abandoned them, and their father felt unable to care for them. He came to visit them in foster placement but avoided answering them when they asked him when they could go home with him. His visit on Saturday had precipitated the current crisis in the foster home. They had been fighting and abusing the 5-year-old daughter of the foster mother.

The occupational therapist decided to conduct her two group assessments at their first session. She started the Draw-A-Person test by placing the boys as far from each other as possible at the primary-sized table. They all drew hurriedly. The two brothers made frequent aggressive comments to each other. While an aide took the boys for a snack, the therapist assembled the materials for the Build-a-City assessment. She had empty thread spools, plasticene modeling clay, tape, glue, construction paper, colored pencils, string, scissors, blunt table knives, wooden clay modeling tools, and styrofoam cubes. She gave them the direction to build an ideal city in 45 minutes. The boys all began to grab items from the table. They worked individually for some minutes. Ronald began to draw and cut out cars. Paul began to draw a house. Tom dropped his own attempt at taping sheets of construction paper together for a street map and grabbed Paul's picture saying, "Let me show you how to make a house." He turned Paul's paper over and folded the sides of the paper to make a three-dimensional rectangle. Then he taped the folds in place and threw it back to Paul saying, "Cut a door and some windows, stupid!" The therapist was tempted to intervene but decided to wait until after the evaluation was over. The hostile interaction between the two brothers soon included Ronald as well. Tom had taken charge and the other two boys chafed under his dictatorial manner, but neither resisted him physically. The completed city consisted of three sheets of gray construction paper taped together. Strips of black paper were glued on top of the gray paper as streets. There were four blue and yellow rectangular paper houses and a red hamburger shop. Tom had made three clay human figures that he stood up between the houses. Ronald's six cars and two trucks were two-dimensional and were propped up on the streets between small balls of clay.

In the discussion following their work, the boys frequently interrupted each other as they tried to explain the importance of each object. Tom invariably won out and explained for the other boys. Ronald was able to demonstrate two cars crashing at a corner and, in the process, squashed one of Tom's clay people. Tom began to hit Ronald, but the therapist intervened and helped them clean up paper scraps. Each boy earned a checkmark for cleaning up. She sent the boys to the dayroom with an aide. Tom and Paul were each assessed individually with the Meeting Street Test. Impulsiveness was their greatest problem.

In the afternoon session, she decided to help the boys make two paper bag puppets each so they could begin to act out their anger and aggression in a structured way. The boys drew eyes, noses, mouths, and other features with felt pens. They pasted paper, yarn, and pieces of cloth for hats and clothes. The next day, each boy was invited to give a puppet show with his two paper bag puppets. By the third puppet show, Tom asked Ronald to help him by handling and being one of his puppets. This was a positive sign of learning to cooperate. The boys were rewarded with checkmarks for improved cooperation. The therapist felt that paper crafts might be used often with the boys during the next week, along with a variety of other activities.

DISCUSSION QUESTIONS

1. What reason would the therapist have for not intervening when the boys verbally abused each other during the Build-a-City assessment?
2. Had the therapist chosen to start the boys out at the second session making papier mâché masks instead of puppets, what kind of problems do you think she might have encountered?
3. It is common for children to make gifts for their parents. What might you suggest to these three boys to make for their parents?

REFERENCES

AOTA Practice Division. (1988). *Mental health information packet.* Rockville, MD: American Occupational Therapy Association.

Barron, D. (1992). *Paper casting: A beginner's guide.* Norcross, GA: Plaid Enterprises, Inc.

Bottomley, J. (1983). *Paper projects for creative kids of all ages.* Boston: Little, Brown and Company.

Department of the Army. (1971). *Craft techniques in occupational therapy,* Washington DC: U.S. Government Printing Office.

Fabri, R. (1966). *Sculpture in paper.* New York: Watson-Guptill Publications.

Gaitskell, C. D., & Hurwitz, A. (1975). *Children and their art* (3rd ed.). New York: Harcourt, Brace, Jovanovitch.

Hainsworth, P. K., & Siqueland, M. L. (1969). *Early identification of children with learning disabilities: The meeting street school screening test.* East Providence, RI: The Easter Seal Society for Crippled Children and Adults of Rhode Island.

Hemphill, B. J. (1982). *The evaluative process in psychiatric occupational therapy.* Thorofare, NJ: SLACK Incorporated.

Llorens, L. A. (1969). An evaluation procedure for children 6-10 years of age. *Am J Occup Ther, 21*(2), 64-69.

Moseley, S., Johnson, P., & Koenig, H. (1962). *Craft designs.* Belmont, CA: Wadsworth.

Reader's Digest. (1979). *Crafts and hobbies.* Pleasantville, NY: Reader's Digest Association, Inc.

Sakade, F. (1958). *Origami: Book two: Japanese paper-folding.* Rutland, VT: Charles E. Tuttle Company.

Titus, J. (1997). Treatment interventions used on level II occupational therapy. Unpublished manuscript.

COOKING AS A CRAFT

INTRODUCTION

The first sentence of this book defines a craft as "an occupation requiring special skill" and a skill as "a learned power of doing a thing competently" (*Webster's Collegiate Dictionary*, 1969). These descriptions obviously put cooking into the craft category. Food, after air and water, is our greatest need. This is undoubtedly one of the reasons there are more cookbooks published than any other category of text and why cooking is the most commonly practiced craft in all occupational therapy clinics. Everyone has to eat.

How did cooking start? Many of us have undoubtedly been raised with Charles Lamb's story about the first roast pig in which the man's house burned and cooked the pig's flesh, which the man then tasted. More probably, the homo erectus were the first primates to cook. Cooking makes food tasty and less tough, and cooked foods keep longer. Perhaps these reasons motivated homo erectus to expand on this craft. First attempts probably were similar to Charles Lamb's tale. Homo erectus may have simply laid a joint of meat on the coals of a fire by mistake, then ran to recover it, tasted it, and said, "yum yum."

Neanderthals apparently developed stews by hanging a skin holding water and meat over a fire. The wet leather would not burn but the heat would boil the stew. Neolithic humans evidently developed the technique of dropping hot stones into a pit of water to cook grains. The development of ceramic pots helped in the refinement of early cooking. Discovery of the properties of metal carried the development of food preparation to an even more skilled level, as did ovens and fireplaces in which heat could be more controlled than in an open fire. This process of improved efficiency continued with development of food preservation, cooking stoves, refrigerators, and on up into the era of microwaves (Beeuwkes, Todhunter, Weigley, 1967; Ritchie, 1981).

Our own cultural background greatly affects what foods we choose. Cultural foods are affected by economics, climate, growing season, geological aspects of soil and water, and food ideas our ancestors brought with them from their native homes (Hames, Joseph, 1986). Often when we crave something in particular, it relates back to early food experiences. For example, to some people peanut butter and graham crackers bring back feelings of childhood mid-morning snack time.

Many people attribute eating problems to early associations with food. Food a person once enjoyed may come to seem like a necessity. They unconsciously desire the former good feeling associated with eating that food and want to achieve it again by repeating the food experience, expecting to get the same emotional experience (Hamilton, Whitney, 1979; Mosey, 1986).

A way to think about food and cooking is to use Maslow's Hierarchy of Human Needs, illustrated in Chapter 8 (see Figure 8-1). Food can be used in an attempt to fulfill the needs expressed at any level. At the lowest level, food and cooking can be for nutrition. At the level of love and belonging, many people associate cooking with a mother's care and family dinners. Success and self-esteem on the next level can be expressed by eating in nice restaurants. On the highest level, many men and women express self-actualization by doing creative cooking. An activity associated with food can appeal to a client functioning at almost any level. Food and cooking can be used to accomplish occupational therapy goals with almost all clients.

FREQUENCY OF USE

Seven out of 10 therapists in clinics use cooking. This craft is used more than any other. It is used to improve bilateral dexterity and encourage self-expression. Mealtimes, eating, and homemaking are also used to increase socialization and improve fine motor control. Nonetheless, cooking traditionally was seldom mentioned in occupational therapy literature (Colson, 1944; Dunton, Licht, 1957; Fidler, Fidler, 1954; Hall, Buck, 1916; Willard, Spackman, 1947). The 1988 *Willard and Spackman's Occupational Therapy* (Hopkins, Smith, 1988) mentions only "dietary considerations" under home management skills and the homemaking evaluation. The most recent edition, 1998, mentions meal preparation as part of evaluation and provides meal preparation guidelines for treatment (Neistadt, Crepeau, 1998). This important craft has had little formal acknowledgment.

ASSESSMENTS

Cooking evaluations have been included as part of occupational therapy homemaking assessments for some time (Williard, Spackman, 1947; Hopkins, Smith, 1978, 1988; Neistadt, Crepeau, 1998; MacDonald, 1960; Trombly, 1983). These evaluations assess capability to perform the physical and mental processes involved in food preparation. A wide variety of homemaker checklists exist. A cooking evaluation was often seen as part of career rehabilitation assessment for the homemaker. Commonly, a woman was asked to prepare a cake mix, tuna salad, or a simple casserole. As men's and women's roles have expanded, evaluating cooking skills has become an important consideration for all adults not living in institutions with communal dining. Perhaps the role changes for both men and women are an underlying cause for cooking being the most used craft activity.

Current evaluations that include cooking as a part of assessment are The Jacobs Prevocational Skills Assessment, The Scoreable Self-Care Evaluation, Instrumental Activities of Daily Living Scale (IADL), Comprehensive Evaluation of Basic Living Skills, the Interest Checklist, and the Street Survival Skills Questionnaire. Food preparation is the last of 15 tasks in the Jacobs Prevocational Skills Assessment. Clients are presented with materials and illustrated instructions for making honey butter and crackers. They are timed and scored on 15 performance areas. They do get to eat the crackers at the end (Jacobs, 1991).

Actual cooking performance is not done in the Scoreable Self-Care Evaluation, but there is a food selection section. It involves choosing and planning menus for all meals for 2 days. The client is scored on whether the menus are nutritionally balanced. For kitchen clean-up, the client is asked to place 10 task cards in sequence.

In IADL, food preparation is one of eight tasks scored for degree of independence. It is an assessment for older adults. The therapist observes the client doing the various tasks and rates performance on a dependence/independence scale (Hemphill, 1988; Kane, Kane, 1985).

On the Comprehensive Evaluation of Basic Living Skills, the client is observed while planning meals, shopping, preparing meals, serving, eating and clean-up, as well as using the telephone and taking a public bus. All components of each task are rated from unable to perform to able to perform independently and correctly (Hemphill, 1988).

The Neuropsychiatric Institute (NPI) Interest Checklist includes barbecues and cooking on its list of 80 activities that clients rate for their interest level. In the discussion following the completion of the list, this can be a stimulator for discussion of leisure choices. Such checklists are used in one in four of all psychiatric occupational therapy departments (Early, 1993). A positive response about cooking on the Interest Checklist will offer an opportunity to persuade a client to participate in a cooking activity in the occupational therapy kitchen.

The Street Survival Skills Questionnaire is a test of adaptive skills in nine basic areas. Domestics is the area that includes 12 questions on cooking. The client is shown pictures and asked questions about food preparation processes related to the pictures. There is a curriculum guide that has lessons to use to teach the areas for which deficits are found (AOTA Practice Division, 1988).

FOOD PROJECTS

The projects presented here are graded from simple to more complex. Most hospitalized clients will hopefully eat food prepared according to these recipes. If there is any doubt about whether a specific client can eat a particular food, consult the client's physician.

Simple Food Project: Stuffed Celery

SUPPLIES

- Washed and trimmed 4-inch stalks of celery
- Non-hydrogenated peanut butter
- Softened cream cheese
- Metal table knife

PROCESS

Since this is a simple one-step process, the therapist will need to have previously washed, trimmed, and cut the celery into 4-inch lengths. The only step for a client is to evenly spread the peanut butter or cheese into the groove in the celery. A second step could be to attractively arrange the stuffed celery on a plate. Food projects as simple as this could be used with young children, with the moderately mentally retarded, or for anyone working on bilateral fine motor activities.

Easy Food Project: Pasta Salad

SUPPLIES

- 8-ounce package of pasta
- 2 cups of cubed cooked meat, such as chicken
- 1 cup of sliced raw vegetables, such as broccoli, celery, carrots, or tomatoes
- 1 cup of salad dressing

EQUIPMENT

- Stove and refrigerator
- 2-quart pot with lid
- 1-cup measuring cups
- 2 sharp cutting knives

- 2 cutting boards
- Drainer
- Large salad bowl
- Serving spoon

PROCESS

1. Cook the pasta according to the directions on the package.
2. Drain, rinse, and allow the pasta to drain again in the drainer.
3. Mix the pasta, meat, and vegetables in a large bowl.
4. Pour the dressing over and stir gently.
5. Chill in the refrigerator.

This recipe makes six servings (Hershey Pasta Group Kitchens, 1985). It may be used as a group cooking project in which one client cooks and rinses the pasta, another cubes the meat, another slices the vegetables, and a fourth mixes the ingredients. It could be served as part of a meal cooked by a group as part of a nutrition or socialization session. Because the process involves potentially dangerous activities—boiling food and cutting with sharp knives—clients need close supervision. If the session is one on a psychiatric unit, a tool count must be completed after dishes are washed and before any clients leave in order to prevent self-injurious incidents.

More Complex Project: Salt-Free Wheat Bread

This bread recipe has no salt, very little sweetening, and almost no cholesterol.

SUPPLIES

- 1 package of dry yeast
- 1/4 cup of lukewarm water
- 1 1/4 cups all-purpose flour
- 1 1/4 cups whole wheat flour
- 2 tablespoons of molasses
- 3/4 cup of lukewarm skim milk
- 2 tablespoons of vegetable oil
- 2 teaspoons margarine or butter

PROCESS

1. Grease the loaf pan with one teaspoon of margarine or butter using the fingers; wash the margarine or butter off the hands (nonstick cooking spray may be substituted).
2. Test the lukewarm water by dropping a drop on the inner wrist to determine if it is at body temperature, which is lukewarm. Stir in the molasses. Sprinkle the yeast over this mixture and stir until it is dissolved. Allow it to stand.

3. Measure the two kinds of flour into a bowl.
4. Mix the flour evenly and make a crater in the middle.
5. Pour the yeast mixture, lukewarm milk, and oil into the crater and mix until the dough is smooth.
6. Turn the dough out onto a counter top that has been dusted with a thin layer of flour.
7. Knead the dough by quickly pressing to flatten it slightly then folding it over, and flattening and folding. Continue this process for 2 minutes. Keep the countertop lightly dusted with flour.
8. Form a ball with the dough.
9. With the other teaspoon of margarine or butter, grease a mixing bowl (or spray it with nonstick cooking spray).
10. Place the dough in the bowl and turn it over to coat it with margarine or butter. Lay a cloth or paper towel over the bowl to protect the dough from drafts of cold air, as well as from dust.
11. Put the bowl in a warm place to allow the dough to rise for 1 hour.
12. Put the dough back on the floured counter and punch it down.
13. Form a loaf shape and place it in the greased pan. Cover it and allow the dough to rise for 45 minutes.
14. Preheat the oven to 350°F.
15. Bake the loaf for 30 minutes.
16. Remove the pan from the oven and place it on a wire rack to cool for 10 minutes.
17. Turn the pan over to get the bread out.

For clients on restricted diets, learning to make their own bread can be very helpful. For people who have allergies to wheat, they can substitute soy or rye flour. To perform this activity adequately, the client needs at least 3 hours, enough sensory reception to be able to determine temperature, follow written or oral directions, keep the tasks in sequence, read numbers, and remember time limits for waiting and baking. A kitchen timer may be helpful for this aspect of the activity. It is possible to bake this loaf in a toaster oven if a 7 x 11-inch rectangular pan is used. If the occupational therapy clinic does not have a kitchen, a toaster oven or microwave oven can offer many cooking possibilities.

MAIN THERAPEUTIC APPLICATIONS

Physical Dysfunction

For the sick person unable to do many things, food often becomes a focus of much attention. If the disability causes a disturbance in the eating process, for example in the case of a stroke, spinal cord injury, or head and neck surgery, helping the client in choosing appropriate foods is an important activity.

Weight control or diabetic diets may be important issues to deal with in using cooking as treatment with clients. Planning meals and practicing cooking can be major activities clients need to do to prove to themselves that they will be able to surmount their problem and continue to enjoy life (Hopkins, Smith, 1983). With neurological clients (such as stroke), cooking can be useful in dealing with safety issues, mobility, balance, and cognitive deficits such as memory, judgment, and sequencing. For the blind, managing in the kitchen, where there are so many possible hazards, is a primary area of treatment concern. There are many aids and adaptive devices for clients who need this kind of help with food preparation. Companies who sell adaptive equipment of this kind are listed in Appendix I.

Mental Health

Because food is so often tied to our early experiences of feeling loved and nurtured, cooking provides a rich opportunity for clients to relearn to nurture themselves. Depressed clients often have little appetite and may be difficult to coax to participate. Sometimes the involvement of a whole group in cooking will draw them in. Special care must be observed with suicidal clients when they are using sharp tools. Manic clients often want to cook elaborate dishes or meals. They may become distracted before they have progressed far with their task. Schizophrenics may be slow about doing the cooking task they are assigned. They will need close supervision, as with all mental health clients. For those who have eating disorders such as anorexia nervosa, bulimia, or obesity, a cooking activity is an opportunity to explore the reasons for the dysfunction such as family dysfunction or early abuse. It is also an opportunity to do a great deal of teaching about nutrition. Those with dementias are particularly prone to mistake one ingredient for another or to even add nonfoods to the mixture. Care must be taken to supervise such clients closely until their functional level is assessed.

Personality-disordered clients, alcoholics, and drug abusers should have little difficulty in most food preparation activities. Meals make a good opportunity to discuss how life without drugs or alcohol will affect their mealtime patterns. The mildly retarded with IQs of 50 to 70 may often live in situations where cooking for themselves is expected. Sometimes they marry and have families. Meal planning, cooking, and clean-up are very important skills to be developed with this population. The moderately retarded with IQs of 35 to 50 may enjoy cooking but need careful supervision. They seldom progress beyond second grade academic skills. Few of these people marry. Often they live in group homes where food needs are filled and no cooking is necessary (APA, 1994; Robinson, Robinson, 1976).

Instructional curricula for food preparation can be purchased from the vendors listed in Appendix I.

Pediatrics

Bonding between infants and adults is most often associated with receiving and giving food. Early play experiences for children often involve playing house, making mud or sand pies, and having tea parties. Early work experiences may involve feeding pets, cleaning up after themselves after meals, or getting their own snack. Children do not often like highly spiced foods. Simple food preparation like stuffing celery or stirring chocolate drink mix into milk may be good for young children. Puppets can be an avenue for children with eating problems who must deal with feelings they have related to their illness (Saunders, 1978). Children 8 to 12 years of age may enjoy making cookies, sandwiches, or preparing frozen pizza. Teenagers often benefit from the complete preparation sequence—making a list, shopping, cooking, eating, and cleaning up. Eating can be a very social time for adolescents who are attempting to decide who they are and what they value. When cooking with children or adolescents, beware of food ending up on the ceiling or walls! Close supervision is recommended (Pratt, Allen, 1989).

Geriatrics

Since most of the elderly are women, and traditionally women have been homemakers and cooks, many elderly clients will have a rich history of cooking from which to draw. Reminiscence groups may elicit accounts of wonderful foods prepared in the past. Actual cooking experiences sometimes elicit involvement from clients whose memory problems keep them from participation in many other activities. Somehow the stimulation of the smell and taste receptors seems to jog memories that appear otherwise unretrievable. Vision problems can interfere with reading recipes, reading package ingredients, and setting oven dials. Hearing difficulties will make bell-type kitchen timers almost useless. Memory problems may cause an elderly person to forget a hot burner. Balance, decreased strength, and arthritis difficulties can make carrying pots and ingredients hazardous. The kitchen is the most common place for accidents to happen. Nonetheless, since cooking and feeding are traditional ways to give of oneself and to oneself, this craft activity has great value for the elderly (Desnick, 1971; Mace, Robins, 1981; Wolff, 1970).

CASE STUDY

Iris is a divorced 56-year-old African-American domestic worker. She was employed by a 35-year-old single mother who was the vice president of a mortgage company. Iris cared for the woman's child as well as her house. In her late 40s, Iris's physician put her on hypertension and cholesterol-lowering drugs. These problems had seemed to be controlled until Iris suffered a left cerebrovascular accident (CVA). After recovering from unconsciousness, she found herself unable to pull herself up off the carpet where she fell. She had to wait for her employer to return from work in the evening before she was discovered. The ambulance took her to the emergency department of a large nearby university teaching hospital. Her employer called her children to meet at the emergency department. It was decided that immediate carotid artery surgery would help prevent further damage. After this procedure, she was placed on the neurointensive care unit.

It was here that the inpatient occupational therapist first evaluated her. He assessed her passive range of motion, active range of motion, muscle tone, strength, oral musculature, visual-motor perception, sensory perception, cognition, and general emotional mood. She was found to have right unilateral paresis in both upper and lower extremities with diminished tactile perception of sharp/dull, hot/cold, position in space, and two-point perception. Her right hand had a very weak grip with some cog wheel jerking as she attempted to move it. Her right leg would buckle under her soon after she got onto her feet. Physical therapy began to work with her in strengthening and range of motion. When the speech therapist tested her oral musculature she had some weakness, though she could achieve lip closure and had no trouble swallowing. The theory underlying treatment in this inpatient clinic was the neuromotor behavior model; consequently, treatment addressed performance deficits as a form of motor behavior, however lifestyle was also a consideration.

In the interview with Iris, the occupational therapist had no difficulty understanding her responses, though her speech was slow and slurred. She labored over each sentence. He found Iris to be rather depressed and worried about her job. Her employer had been paying her health insurance. She feared that her employer would find another domestic worker before Iris recovered and that she might lose her health insurance benefits as well as her job, which she liked better than any domestic job she had held before. She was unaware of the COBRA law regarding insurance continuance. The pay was good compared to other domestic worker's pay and her employer was concerned about her welfare. The occupational therapist told Iris he would send the case manager to help her with these issues. Iris's daughter rearranged her schedule to partially take over her mother's job while she was in the hospital. The occupational therapist and Iris discussed a kitchen evaluation to see how much she could actually do.

On the second day after the carotid surgery, Iris was moved out of neurointensive care onto the medical floor. At this time, the certified occupational therapy assistant (COTA) took her in a wheelchair to the occupational therapy kitchen for a screening. First the COTA showed her where things were in the kitchen. She showed Iris how easily she could roll the wheelchair up to the sink and countertop stove in the adapted kitchen. Iris slowly told her that the kitchen of her employer had high countertops and a microwave over the stove. The COTA reassured her that she would probably have more recovery before she went back to work. Indeed, it did appear that Iris had begun to have some recovery in her right hand, though her leg still buckled under her. In the kitchen evaluation, the COTA asked Iris to start by making a tuna sandwich. Iris was able to wash a celery stalk but had trouble trimming it before she put it in the food processor. She had difficulty using the electric can opener. The COTA showed her several helpful techniques, such as holding the bowl in her lap for mixing and using a rimmed cutting board for spreading the tuna salad on the bread.

As they worked together, Iris began to talk about her job and family life. She told of occasions when her employer had guests, of how she often made and served elaborate six-course meals. Often on these evenings, she stayed overnight at her employer's home. Her own children were grown, though two still lived with her in her little house. Iris described her job as interesting and fulfilling. She had been a domestic worker most of her adult life.

She had worked 5 years in her present job, and it had been the best job she'd ever had. She'd never felt as much a part of a family for whom she worked as she had on her current job. Her main goal, as she expressed it, was to get back to work.

After the COTA and occupational therapist had a chance to discuss her various evaluations, they decided she would probably benefit from having all her therapy in the occupational therapy kitchen. Her sessions were scheduled at 11:30 am, and the kitchen staff was instructed to send a tray of raw food that Iris would prepare for herself after her exercises. In the occupational therapy kitchen, everything could be reached from the wheelchair, though Iris was increasingly able to pull herself up to standing if necessary. Using the over-the-sink paring board, Iris made vegetable salad, cut vegetables for a casserole, and sliced fruit for gelatin salad. By the end of the second week, she was almost independent in preparing her lunch.

At this time, she was transferred to the rehabilitation center in the same hospital complex in which Rehabilitation Theory was used. Close communication between the two occupational therapy departments made it possible for the rehabilitation occupational therapist to make a smooth transition for Iris. During her 3 weeks in the rehabilitation hospital, she learned how to use many new pieces of adaptive equipment such as a reacher, a one-handed can opener, a jar opener, a miracle peeler, and a Swedish knife for those with weak grip. Her strength in her right hand had gradually shown improvement but was still not fully recovered. With the special Swedish knife, she was able to do almost all the cutting she needed. On her last session before being discharged, Iris cooked a meal for the occupational therapy staff as her way of saying thank you. She made oven-barbecued ribs, field peas, turnip greens, and corn bread. The only assistance she needed was with shelling the peas. She got a paraplegic client to help her with that, as she still had problems with some fine motor activities. The occupational therapy staff helped her serve the meal. Most of Iris's initial depression was gone, and on this occasion it was not evident at all.

Iris started back to her job on a part-time basis. She moved into the guestroom at her employer's house so she would not have to immediately deal with taking the city bus. Initially, she just cooked the evening meal and supervised the child when she returned from school. At the end of 7 months, Iris was working full-time again.

DISCUSSION QUESTIONS

1. If the CVA victim was a male laborer instead of Iris, how could cooking be adapted to appeal to him?
2. If a member of a cooking group has special dietary needs, such as salt-free meals or a strict diabetic diet, how could you adapt meal planning and cooking of spaghetti to fill his or her needs?
3. Clients taking the antidepressant drug called *MAO inhibitors* are prohibited from eating the following foods because they could cause a hypertensive crisis: beans, aged cheese, yeast, beer, liquor, wine, yogurt, liver, and pickled herring. Plan a menu and choose recipes safe for such a client.

REFERENCES

American Psychiatric Association. (1994). *Diagnotic and statistical manual of mental disorders* (4th ed.). Washington, DC: American Psychiatric Association.

AOTA Practice Division. (1988). *Mental health information packet.* Rockville, MD: American Occupational Therapy Association.

Beeuwkes, A. M., Todhunter, E .H., & Weigley, E. S. (eds). (1967). *Essays on history of nutrition and dietetics.* Chicago: The American Dietetics Association.

Colson, J. H. C. (1944). *The rehabilitation of the injured: Occupational therapy.* London, Cassell and Company.

Desnick, S. G. (1971). *Geriatric contentment.* Springfield, IL: Charles C. Thomas.

Dunton, W. R., & Licht, S. (1957). *Occupational therapy principles and practice.* Springfield, IL: Charles C. Thomas.

Early, M. B. (1993). *Mental health concepts and techniques for the occupational therapy assistant* (2nd ed.). New York: Raven Press.

Fidler, G. S., & Fidler, J. W. (1954). *Introduction to psychiatric occupational therapy.* New York: the MacMillan Co.

Hall, H. J., & Buck, M. M. C. (1916). *Handicrafts for the handicapped.* New York: Moffat, Yard and Co.

Hames, C. C., & Joseph, D. H. (1986). *Basic concepts of helping: A holistic approach* (2nd ed.). Norwalk, CT: Appleton-Century-Crofts.

Hamilton, E. M., & Whitney, E. (1979). *Nutrition concepts and controversies.* St. Paul, MN: West Publishing Company.

Hemphill, B. J. (1988). *Mental health assessment in occupational therapy.* Thorofare, NJ: SLACK Incorporated.

Hershey Pasta Group Kitchens. (1985). *The Hurry Up I'm Hungry Pasta Cookbook.* Hershey, PA: Hershey Foods Corporation.

Hopkins, H. L., & Smith, H. D. (1978). *Willard and Spackman's occupational therapy* (5th ed.). Philadelphia: Lippincott.

Hopkins, H. L., & Smith, H. D. (1983). *Willard and Spackman's occupational therapy* (6th ed.). Philadelphia: Lippincott.

Hopkins, H. L., & Smith H. D. (1988). *Willard and Spackman's occupational therapy* (7th ed.). Philadelphia: Lippincott.

Jacobs, K. (1991). *Occupational therapy: Work-related programs and assessments* (2nd ed.). Boston: Little, Brown and Company.

Kane, R. A., & Kane, R. L. (1985). *Assessing the elderly: a practical guide to measurement.* Lexington, MA: Lexington Books.

MacDonald, E. M. (1960). *Occupational therapy in rehabilitation.* London: Bailliere, Tindall and Cox.

Mace, N. L., & Robins, P. V. (1981). *The 36-hour day.* Baltimore: Johns Hopkins University Press.

Mosey, A. C. (1986). *Psychosocial components of occupational therapy,* New York: Raven Press.

Neistadt, M. E., & Crepeau, E. B. (1998). *Willard and Spackman's occupational therapy.* Philadelphia: Lippincott.

Pratt, P. N., & Allen, A. S. (1989.) *Occupational therapy for children* (2nd ed.). St. Louis: Mosby.

Ritchie, C. I. A. (1981). *Food in civilization.* Sydney, Australia: Methuen Australia Pty., Ltd.

Robinson, N. M., & Robinson, H. B. (1976). *The mentally retarded child: A psychological approach.* New York: McGraw-Hill.

Saunders, F. M. (1978). *Your diabetic child.* New York: Bantam books.

Trombly, C. A. (1983). *Occupational therapy for physical dysfunction* (2nd ed.). Baltimore: Waverly Pres.

Webster's Seventh New Collegiate Dictionary. (1969). Springfield, MA: G & C Merriam Company.

Willard, H. S., & Spackman, C. E. (1947). *Principles of occupational therapy.* Philadelphia: Lippincott.

Wolff, K. (1970). *The emotional rehabilitation of the geriatric patient.* Springfield, IL: Charles C. Thomas.

COMPUTER ART AS A CRAFT

INTRODUCTION

Initially, it is important to say what this chapter is not. It is not going to tell you how to buy a computer, what kind to buy, how to use it, how to speak computerese/computer jargon, or what the computer's potential for total client treatment could be. There are already some good books about this (Anson, 1996; Cook, Hussey, 1995; Pomeroy, 1997; Clark, 1986; Cromwell, 1986; McWilliams, 1984; AOTA Practice Division, 1985, 1994; Ryan, 1986). Remember, though, that the computer field, like all technologies, is constantly being improved and refined.

It is hard to pinpoint the first computer. Some say it was the abacus, which is 2500 years old (Pascoe, 1974). Others say it was a primitive slide-rule type machine invented in Germany in 1623 (Ritchie, 1986). In this century, B.F. Skinner, the American father of behavioral therapy and teaching machines, has been given credit as a pioneer in this field. His 1953 effort to help his daughter learn arithmetic with a machine using cards, levers, and lights may have been the grandparent of today's modern computer graphics (Hall, 1983).

In occupational therapy, the first articles on computers and occupational therapy appeared in the 1960s (AOTA Practice Division, 1985). The 1975 article in *The American Journal of Occupational Therapy,* "Computers and Occupational Therapy," mentions art and recreation as possible therapy tools. Some prognosticators anticipated that everyone would be a graphics user by the beginning of the new century (Hallisey, 1989). Since only 40% of U.S. citizens have access to computers according to a government study, it appears those predictions are ambitious. However, just as crafts cannot be replaced, computers will not eliminate our other treatment modalities. They are just additional tools (AOTA Practice Division, 1985, 1994).

Bedside computer work stations for acute care hospitals are being used in many places. Their primary purpose is for record keeping and documentation of the client's condition. However, if a bedside terminal is available, therapists can use it for client treatment. Therapists need to check with their computer department before loading graphics or any software on a network computer system. It could be possible for the software loaded at a workstation to conflict with the operation of the computer in a networked environment. If the therapist receives permission to load such software, the graphics craft would be used in the same way in which a therapist sometimes allows clients to continue to work on an occupational therapy project on their own after the therapist has gone. Clients might be allowed to keep computer software and work on it at their leisure (AOTA, 1988).

In the same developmental progression that makes children naturally draw before they write, most adults can use graphics before learning word processing. Many graphics software packages make simple lines and shapes that are the first marks, besides scribbles, that children make when they begin to handle pencils and crayons. Other software allows the user to simply color in existing pictures. Software programs are on a square plastic disk or round compact disk. Most new computers on the market today have a drawing program already installed. When a person, (even a therapist) first attempts to draw using a mouse, which is the usual hand control for graphics, it is similar to the experience a child has when first starting to use traditional writing implements. The mouse responds to the user's untrained hand in which a tiny muscle contraction sends the pencil cursor on the screen streaking off in an unintended direction.

Some clients may have or will develop more skill and creative possibilities with graphics software while others may benefit from and enjoy programs in which pictures are pre-drawn. The client needs only to choose the picture, which can then be rotated, stretched, or changed in size. The wide spectrum of available graphics software makes it possible to easily grade the activity up or down. Computer graphics are similar to painting, in which for some clients paint-by-number is appropriate and for others oil paint motivates them to create. Truly, computer art can be a helpful craft for clients who think of themselves as being a part of our modern computer age. Other arts, such as poetry writing, music composition, and arrangement can be done on the computer. The idea of creating with this technology can be quite motivating for some clients.

FREQUENCY OF USE

Many clinics have computers that can be made available for client treatment. While most clinics use their computers for record keeping and cognitive evaluations, the use of computers for treatment is becoming more commonplace. Therapists choose computers to accomplish various treatment objectives: to improve cognition, increase fine motor control, and encourage self-expression. As more clinics acquire computers and computer expertise, possibilities for treatment activities multiply.

ASSESSMENTS

Computer assessments in occupational therapy include various kinds of evaluations, not all of which are graphic. *Graphic* means pictorial arts or clear visual images. Cognitive dysfunction, which includes attention deficits, memory problems, confusion, lack of comprehension and judgment, spatial disorientation, and decreased ability to solve problems is one of the areas most often evaluated using computers.

Graphics are used in evaluation of head-injured and learning disabled clients (Milner, 1984). Initially, clients must be evaluated for appropriateness of computer assessment. Can they see the screen well enough? There are compensating strategies for people who have trouble seeing the screen. Screen enlargement programs, such as *Zoom Text*, are available that will enlarge anything that is on the screen; however, the client would not be able to see the entire screen without scrolling, just the enlarged area. Can they manipulate the input devices (keyboards, joy sticks, mice, light pens, etc.) to give commands to the computer? Can they comprehend the instructions and questions asked by the computer? Graphics can be used to evaluate clients for vocational appropriateness for drafting or similar careers (Milner, 1984). A game called *Gremlin Hunt* can be used for assessment in head injury and with the developmentally disabled. The graphics are attractive, colorful, and appropriate for clients 8 years of age and up (Timm, 1989). For clients with perceptual problems, *Visual Organization* software evaluates figure ground and visual closure (Redding, 1991). Early and advanced switch games can be used in either treatment or evaluation of using graphics to complete pictures, match shapes and colors, and for directionality, motor control, and praxis. The early games are for children up through 6th grade. The advanced games are for people up through 10th grade (Dilly, 1990). *Colors & Shapes* is an assessment game using color graphics for children 3 to 5 years old. The game comes on three disks: one to assess color discrimination, one to assess shape discrimination, and one for the two skills combined. It is sequenced and the child gets immediate feedback (Loebl, 1993).

The computer is absolutely objective and cannot be manipulated as a therapist can. This can be valuable in evaluating some kinds of clients.

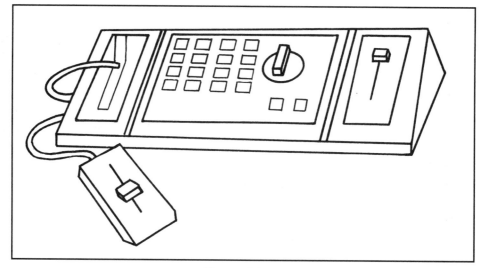

Figure 16-1.
Paddle control board.

MAIN THERAPEUTIC APPLICATIONS

Physical Dysfunction

There are some devices that help the physically disabled client do computer graphics. A joystick is a hand-operated stick control that can move the cursor over the screen to give commands. A light-pencil control can be used by aiming the lighted end of the pencil on the screen to give commands. Another aid is the paddle control used in computer games. A paddle control is a board, usually with two hand-held switches that control the action on the screen for two-player games such as tennis, hockey, and squash (Figure 16-1). These games use graphics or pictures rather than words. Such controls allow clients with severely restricted upper extremity and body movements to control the pictures on the screen. Some games and graphics can be slowed for the restricted user (Clark, 1986). Clients with physical problems who could benefit from computer craft are those who suffer from spinal cord injury, multiple sclerosis, and Guillian-Barres. They can use these games to increase motor control.

As with assessment, those physically dysfunctional clients with cognitive problems are often good candidates for use of computer graphics in treatment. These clients may have acquired their cognitive deficits from many different causes, such as developmental problems, cerebrovascular accident, head injury, cerebral palsy, or learning disabilities (Gracey, 1984; Skinner, Trachtman, 1985).

Mental Health

High-functioning clients can benefit from working with innovative graphics. There are a variety of programs available (*Sax Arts & Crafts Catalog*, 1998). Concentration, attention span, and fatigue, which are frequent problems for depressed clients, could all be addressed through this medium. Manic clients would need precautions, as their hyperactivity, impatience, and poor impulse control could make this activity frustrating. Also, they could damage expensive hardware with their excessive movement. This should only be used with clients who have been stabilized on psychotropic medication. Cognition, such as thinking and problem solving, may be difficult activities for some schizophrenics. A schizophrenic client who could benefit might be in a daycare or sheltered workshop program but would unlikely be found in more acute treatment situations.

Clients with personality disorders may find computer work appealing, as their cognitive integration and perceptual processing functions are usually intact (unless they have been damaged through trauma or abuse of drugs or alcohol). Few mentally retarded have the creative capacity to use the more sophisticated drawing programs; however, the higher-functioning retarded clients may enjoy the programs with pre-drawn pictures. Some of the children's shape and design programs could be helpful in working with the mentally retarded. The therapist would need to be careful that such graphics were not perceived as "kid stuff" by the retarded person, thus making the graphics not age appropriate or demeaning to the retarded client. In all cases, the success of using graphics would be volitional. Motivation for using the computer may be the single most important reason to use it with psychiatric clients (Loebl, 1993).

Pediatrics

Pediatric clients may be the best candidates for computer treatment, as they often have already been exposed to computers if they are of school age (Levin, 1985). They do not have the inherent fear and mental block about new technology that older clients often have. Originally, there had been fears that computer use by children would cause them to fail to develop social skills and to become withdrawn. This appears to have been an exaggerated alarm. Children have grown up being constantly exposed to television and apparently have learned to be perceptive of what comes on the screen in a way that older people have not. Consequently, they are often more able to learn from designs and pictures on a computer monitor, which resembles a television screen, than older clients. An added benefit is that computers give immediate, nonjudgmental, reliable feedback to children about their actions and behavior. Computers cannot be manipulated as adult humans can.

Geriatrics

This client population may be least likely to benefit from computer graphics. Many elders have slowed in their thought processes and movements. The very basis of computing is speed and efficiency, the opposite of what many elders want to do. They want to be allowed to move and think more slowly. In our culture, we allow them that prerogative.

Diminished eyesight is often a problem for geriatric clients. Computer screens are sometimes difficult to visually focus on for more than a few minutes. While we may get the occasional alert older client who is used to operating a computer, it is less common than in other client groups. Graphics may be a difficult new challenge for an elderly client. Programs such as *Zoom Text* are available to compensate for lack of visual acuity.

O'Leary, Mann, and Perkash (1991) discuss problems older people may have with the use of computers and offer some solutions related to positioning, vision, strength, and cognition. They provide an extensive list of resources for adaptive computer equipment. Computer resources for elders continue to be developed (Larson, Stevens-Ratch, Pedretti, Crabtree, 1996).

CASE STUDY

Emily is a 10-year-old severely contracted cerebral palsy client. It was unknown until she was 8 years old that she had an IQ of 110. Because she was so physically handicapped and her language was limited, and because there was no one trained to test her IQ by non-pencil-and-paper methods before, it was thought that she was retarded as well as physically limited. Emily is of African-American and Puerto Rican heritage and was born in New York City. At age 2 1/2 years, she and her mother moved back to her mother's home in the South. Shortly thereafter, her mother, who had been a drug addict, died of an overdose. Emily was taken to live with her grandmother in a rural community. She had had no schooling except what she saw on television. When Emily was 8, her grandmother died and no one else in the family was willing to care for Emily, as she required total personal care, feeding, diapering, and bathing.

The state child welfare agency made a decision to place her in an intermediate care facility for the developmentally disabled. She was finally evaluated and measured for her own wheelchair. At this time she was enrolled in a special education class. All the members of the treatment team evaluated her. At that time, her IQ was discovered to be 110. A concerted effort was made by all the professionals involved with Emily to help her make up for the time she was without schooling. They were assisted by the state assistive technology reference guide (Thompson, Bethea, Rizer, Hutto, 1998). The occupational therapist used a combination of theories, including Learning/Cognitive Disabilities and the Model of Human Occupation. Emily's upper extremity athetosis made most occupational activities difficult for her. The occupational therapy goals were to:

- Increase self-care such as self-feeding, learning to sit on the toilet, and control the timing of toileting
- Learn visual and perceptual motor performance skills
- Enhance and stimulate visual acuity
- Improve upper extremity fine motor coordination and dexterity
- Utilize her motivation to learn to overcome performance deficits
- Develop a feeling of independence and autonomy

She was evaluated for appropriateness of computer use. The therapist found that Emily could begin to control the screen by using a joy stick on her wheelchair lap board. The schoolteacher working with Emily began a program to teach her to read. She had taught herself some words by simply watching television. While attending occupational therapy, she worked with the computer graphics as a reward for feeding herself and waiting to sit on the toilet to urinate and defecate. She started out with a simple program of lines and shapes that she could color in and move around the screen. But she rapidly advanced to a more sophisticated program involving assembling designs on the screen. The therapist worked with her on visually scanning her work, developing figure ground perception by seeing shapes within shapes and figures, on color discrimination and sequencing her actions to get the effects she wanted, and from there to drawing and painting on more sophisticated software. The occupational therapy clinic did not have a color printer so the therapist sent her floppy disk to the curriculum center at the board of education building to have the graphics printed out from Emily's drawings. Soon Emily was skilled enough to draw her own cartoons, which she used on greeting cards.

The school staff used her enlarged cartoons for signs and warnings around the school building. Emily was seen as a good candidate for a new group home for the disabled that was going to be funded by a grant. The occupational therapist worked with the grant writers to see that money was included to buy computers for each resident's room.

DISCUSSION QUESTIONS

1. How could the possibility of increasing Emily's social isolation be avoided as she became more involved with the computer?
2. Could any of the movements she learned to make with the joystick be transferred over to help her in increasing her independence in self-care?

REFERENCES

American Occupational Therapy Association. (1988). In focus. *Am J Occup Ther, 42*(1), 43-47.

Anson, D. K. (1996). *Alternative computer access: A guide to selection.* Philadelphia: F. A. Davis Company.

AOTA Practice Division. (1985). *Computer information packet.* Rockville, MD: American Occupational Therapy Association.

AOTA Practice Division. (1994). *Computers: AOTA resource guide.* Bethesda, MD: American Occupational therapy Association.

Clark, E. N. (1986). *Microcomputer: Clinical applications.* Thorofare, NJ: SLACK Incorporated.

Cook, A. M., & Hussey, S. M (1995). *Assistive technologies: Principles and practices.* St. Louis: Mosby

Cromwell, F .S. (1986). *Computer applications in occupational therapy. New York: The Howarth Press.*

Dilly, S. K. (1990). Software & technology reviews. *American Occupational Therapy Association, 44*(2), 179.

English, C. B. (1973). Computers and occupational therapy. *Am J Occup Ther, 29*(1), 43-47.

Gracey, S. (1984). Computer assisted therapy for brain injured patients: a team approach. *Physical disabilities special interest section newsletter, 7*(2), 4.

Hall, E. (1983). A cure for American education. *Psychology Today, 17*(9), 26-27.

Hallisey, J. (1989). The future is graphic. *PC Computing, 7*(2), 52.

Larson, K. O., Stevens-Ratch, R. G., Pedretti, L., & Crabtree, J. L. (eds.). (1996). *ROTE: The role of OT with the elderly.* Bethesda, MD: American Occupational Therapy Association.

Levin, G. (1985). Computers and kids: the good news. *Psychology Today, 19*(8), 50-51.

Loebl, D. (1993). Colors & Shapes: A computer-based assessment and remediation tool for children's cognitive and perceptual skills. *Isreal Journal of Occupational Therapy. 2*(2), E53-E59.

McWilliams, P. (1984). *Personal computers and the disabled.* Garden City, NY: Doubleday and Company.

Milner, D. (1984). Use of a microcomputer in treatment of patients with physical disabilities. *Physical disabilities special interest section newsletter, 7*(2):1-3.

O'Leary, S., Mann, C., & Perkash, I. (1991). Access to computers for older adults: Problems and solutions. *Am J Occup Ther, 45*(7), 636-642.

Pascoe, L. C. (1974). *Encyclopedia of dates and events.* Kent, United Kingdom: Hadder and Stroughton, Ltd.

Pomeroy, B. (1997). *Beginnernet in rehabilitation: A beginner's guide to the internet and the world wide web.* Thorofare, NJ: SLACK Incorporated

Redding, K. (1991). Software & technology reviews. *Am J Occup Ther, 45*(6), 569-570.

Ritchie, D. (1986). *The computer pioneers: The making of the modern computer,* New York: Simon and Schuster.

Ryan, S. (ed.). (1986). *The certified occupational therapy assistant: Roles and responsibilities.* Thorofare, NJ: SLACK Incorporated.

Sax Arts & Crafts Catalog. (1998.) New Berlin, WI: Sax Arts & Crafts.

Skinner, A. D., & Trachtman, L. H. (1985). Brief or new: use of the computer program (PC coloring book in cognitive rehabilitation). *Am J Occup Ther, 39*(7).

Thompson, A. R., Bethea, L. L., Rizer, H. F., and Hutto, M. D. (1998). *Students with disabilities and assistive technology: A desk reference guide.* Jackson, MS: Mississippi Department of Rehabilitation Services/Project START.

Timm, J. (1989). Software & technology reviews. *Am J Occup Ther. 43*(4), 267.

ART TECHNIQUES, DRAWING, AND PAINTING

INTRODUCTION

Drawing may be the oldest craft used for healing (that we know about). While the crafts discussed so far in this book may be old, it was not until the last few centuries that they have been used in healing. Drawing has been used for millennia in healing practices and other rituals that attempt to control nature (Janson, 1969; Janson, 1995; Lewin, 1988).

Before humans had any knowledge of anatomy and physiology, images conceived in the brain and drawn on a wall were considered as real as any other product, such as a slingshot, and were believed to have as much real power. Images were integral in both killing and healing rituals. The Greeks carried on these practices in the temples of Aesculapias. However, the 17th century French philosopher René Descarte emphasized the mind-body split. This reinforced a direction in which medicine was already headed: the mind and body were separate and needed different healing treatments. Emotions did not qualify as having any relation to disease (Achterberg, 1985).

In 19th century Switzerland, the force of imagery began to be studied in earnest by psychologists. Sigmund Freud was aware of the power of imagery in treatment, though he seldom used it himself (Kaplan, Sadock, 1981, 1998). Florence Goodenough published her work on drawing as an intelligence test in 1926. Art therapy began to develop in the early 1900s—in the same era that occupational therapy had its start (Detre, et al, 1983; Ulman, Dachinger, 1975). Art therapists specialized in using art in healing. Occupational therapists have used drawing in the same way they used so many other activities, when it was the best activity to help rehabilitate a client to functioning most independently. The first edition of Willard and Spackman's *Principles of Occupational Therapy* (1947) has a section on drawing and sketching in treatment. It focuses on both physical and mental, as well as pediatric, uses of art. About this same time, those researching the meaning of drawings began to publish their findings (Betensky, 1973; Hammer, 1958; Harris, 1963; Machover, 1949). While drawing and painting have never been the major modalities in occupational therapy as they are in art therapy, occupational therapists have felt free to use these activities when they were the best ones for the client. These are important techniques for occupational therapists to keep in their armamentarium of treatment tools.

FREQUENCY OF USE

Fingerpainting is used in many clinics. Fingerpainting is used to provide an outlet for frustration, to encourage self-expression, to increase sensory input, and to improve bilateral integration and dexterity. Painting with watercolors, acrylics, or oils is an activity often used to improve fine motor control and eye-hand coordination. Drawing with pencils or crayons occurs in almost half the clinics, particularly those dealing with mental health and cognition. Drawing is often used to improve group socialization, to improve fine motor control, to encourage self-expression, and to improve self-concept.

ASSESSMENTS

There are more drawing assessments than any other craft or art media. Perhaps this is because it is so simple to ask for a drawing that requires few materials and that can be done almost anywhere with individuals or groups. Drawing is adaptable to almost any assessment situation. Many of the assessments mentioned here were developed by occupational therapists in the 1960s and 1970s when the profession was concentrating on standardizing administration, observations, and analyses of task behavior. The first three described below are often used by other professions as well, such as psychology. Perhaps the House-Tree-Person test is one of the earliest drawing assessments that is still used (Buck, 1948). Except for the standard request to draw a house, a tree, and a person on 8 1/2 x 11-inch white paper, this is an unstructured test. The order of drawing is theorized to move from the least threatening (the house), to most threatening symbol (the person). There are guidelines for interpreting each drawing (Oster, Gould, 1987).

The Goodenough-Harris Drawing Test is for children ages 3 to 15 years and can be used individually or in a group. The children are asked to draw first a man, then a woman, and last themselves. There is a scoring guide that tells how to look at each separate item: head, neck, nose, etc. The scores show the child's functioning in relation to age performance expectations (Harris, 1963; Ascher, 1996).

The Draw-a-Person Catalog for Interpretive Analysis is unstructured (Urband, 1963). Clients are simply told to draw a person any way they like. The picture is discussed afterward with the therapist. The catalog has lists of warnings and abnormality indicators for body parts as well as drawing quality. There are a number of checklist forms to assist in documenting the assessment.

The Azima Battery, which was first developed in the late 1950s and early 1960s, includes a free or unstructured drawing, a drawing of a person of the same and opposite sex, an unstructured clay project, and fingerpainting. It is for use in psychiatric occupational therapy. It is intended to assess awareness of reality, perceptions of others, mood, energy level, and ego defenses (Hemphill, 1982a).

The Diagnostic Test Battery has five tasks: drawing, ceramics, painting, woodwork, and leather. It was intended to be for adult psychiatric clients. The House-Tree-Person test is used for the drawing portion. The painting part of the test is an unstructured watercolor. Assessment findings should be expected to include expressiveness, compulsiveness, cognitive processes, mood, and approach to task (Androes, Dreyfus, Bloesch, 1965).

The Fidler Diagnostic Battery was developed in the early 1960s for use with individual clients. It included drawing, fingerpainting, and working with clay. This was refined and developed into the Activity Laboratory that could be used with groups of clients. The Activity Laboratory also has three activities: cutting out and coloring a stencil, fingerpainting, and assembling a collage. The sequence from structured to unstructured tasks is intended to demonstrate how the client deals with limits. The group setting helps assess social skills. Fine motor performance is also observed (Hemphill, 1982a).

The O'Kane Diagnostic Battery for Psychiatry is projective in nature. There are three charcoal drawings, three fingerpaintings, and a clay project. The administration is structured (AOTA Practice Division, 1988).

The Kinetic Family Drawing is normed for ages 5 to 20 years. Clients are simply asked to draw the people in their family. The manual has pictures of client drawings and discussion of a wide variety of symbols and situations. Some therapists incorporate a more informal version of this assessment into a battery of other evaluations in pediatric psychiatry (Burns, Kaufman, 1972).

The Goodman Battery includes a free or unstructured drawing, a drawing of a person along with a tile task, and clay work. This assessment looks at approach to task, effect, impulsiveness, compulsiveness, organization, and symbolic content. It is for adolescents and adults (Hemphill, 1982a).

The Copy Flower House Test is a subjective assessment that is included in a battery for evaluating a variety of perceptual problems experienced by stroke clients. Unilateral neglect is specifically assessed by the two drawings of a flower and a house. Informal person drawings are also helpful in working with clients who have suffered a cerebrovascular accident (CVA) for evaluation of body visualization and somatognosia (Siev, Frieshtat, 1976).

The Bay Area Functional Performance Evaluation (BaFPE) for psychiatry, for clients aged 16 years and older, has five tasks and an assessment of the client's social skills. The five tasks are shell sorting, check depositing, drawing a house plan, arranging a block pattern, and drawing a person doing something. This test is well-validated and, though scoring is initially difficult to learn, it provides good data on dysfunctional areas. Research continues on the BaFPE. It has been revised several times since its introduction in 1978-1979 (AOTA Practice Division, 1988).

The BH Battery has a tile task and fingerpainting. While the materials arrangement is structured, the instructions to the client for painting are not. The client is timed, and the manual provides a rating scale for each activity. Documentation for this assessment is oriented toward behavioral description rather than content analysis (Hemphill, 1982b).

In the Mattis' Dementia Rating Scale, clients are asked to draw a self-portrait, a picture of a person sitting across from them, a face, a house, and a simple still life of arranged objects. This evaluation, developed by an art therapist, is used in helping diagnose perceptual deficits such as figure collision and confusion, which may indicate dementia (Wald, 1983).

The Gross Activity Battery has three projective activities: charcoal drawing, fingerpainting, and working with clay. The administration is highly structured, as is the way in which it is reported. It can be used with any age or client population (AOTA Practice Division, 1988).

The Elizur Test of Psycho-Organicity: Children and Adults is a 10-minute test for individuals aged 6 years and up. The purpose is to differentiate clients with organic brain problems from those without. The test uses drawings, digits, and blocks (AOTA Practice Division, 1988).

Many checklists of leisure preference, such as the Neuropsychiatric Interest (NPI) Checklist, include painting or drawing. These sorts of art techniques offer good potential for leisure activities for many people (Early, 1993). A person does not have to be an artist to enjoy making art.

Supplies

It is not necessary to have an elaborate supply of art materials to be successful in using drawing and painting for crafts. The following materials and supplies are adequate for most clinics.

Twelve x 18-inch paper is best for most art projects as it allows enough room to draw freely without taking up too much table space. The following types should be kept available for artwork.

- Newsprint paper—12 x 18 inches
- White drawing paper—12 x 18 inches
- Manila paper—12 x 18 inches
- Fingerpaint paper—16 x 22 inches

Clients can share boxes of crayons and pens, thus increasing social skills while requiring fewer individual sets of colors.

- #2 pencils with erasers
- Crayons
- Chalk or chalk pastels
- Oil pastels
- Felt-tip markers
- Powdered tempera paint (this can be mixed with dish detergent and water to make fingerpaint)
- Boxes of watercolors with semi-moist half pans
- An assortment of brushes

In special instances, oil paints may be desirable for clients who are artists. Otherwise, watercolor or tempera is adequate for most painting projects.

DRAWING AND PAINTING

There is such a vast array of techniques for using painting and drawing in therapy that the development of a separate profession, art therapy, was natural in the same way that the diversity of plant-growing techniques made horticulture therapy natural. Occupational therapy incorporates aspects of both drawing and painting into treatment when the situation indicates (Liebman, 1986; Rhyne, 1973; Robbins, Sibley, 1976). Apart from the evaluations discussed before, occupational therapists use many art media to achieve client goals. Several are described below.

Murals

Murals are a way of using art to achieve a group goal. A mural can be drawn with crayons or painted with tempera paint. They can be done on brown butcher paper, on glass windows at holidays, or on newsprint. Sometimes newspaper publishers have the ends of rolls of newsprint that they cannot use and may be willing to donate. This paper is good for group murals. Painting on windows is fun until it is time to clean them off. The work involved in removal can be minimized by adding liquid detergent to the tempera paints when mixing them. Liquid dish detergent added to tempera paint gives a nice consistency to the paint as well as allowing it to wash out of clothing more easily. Damp rags will often remove this paint from windows with less effort. If brown butcher paper is used, tempera paint is bright enough to overcome the darkness of the brown background. It is difficult to make crayon show up on brown butcher paper. It is better to use bright felt markers on it instead if drawing is to be used rather than painting. Care must be taken with permanent markers, as the fumes can be toxic. Be sure the area is well-ventilated and the client does not inhale these fumes for any length of time (Anonymous, 1986).

Crayon Resist

This technique elevates crayons to a more sophisticated level for most clients.

PROCESS

1. Using 12 x 18-inch manila paper, have the client draw a crayon design or picture with white or pale pastel colors.
2. Put one drop of water in the half-pan of watercolor to be used. Allow the water to soften the color for a few minutes. It is better to use a bright vivid color to contrast with the crayon.
3. Dip the brush into the water and stroke the top of the watercolor half-pan to gather color into the brush. Then apply the watercolor to the whole sheet.
4. Repeat the softening process if necessary. This technique makes attractive snow scenes.

Crayon Etching

Crayon etching is a more difficult technique and requires physical effort and endurance but usually produces an attractive product. Use paper with a tooth, which means it has a slightly rough surface, such as construction or manila paper. It may be best to start with a smaller size at first, such as 8 1/2 x 11 inches.

PROCESS

1. Heavily color all areas of the paper with different colors. It works well if the colors are in contrasting sections. Color heavily to make sure none of the paper shows through.
2. Use a black crayon to completely cover all the other colors.
3. When no color shows through the black, use a sharp instrument like the pointed end of a leather tracing modeler to scratch a picture through the black crayon.

This activity can use up a lot of energy and aggression because of the effort involved in coloring then scratching through the surface. This classifies as a constructive/destructive craft in which a client can sublimate negative impulses. This kind of activity/occupation can use motions that simulate destructive force at the same time the client is creating.

MAIN THERAPEUTIC APPLICATIONS

Physical Dysfunction

Fingerpainting may be used with a client who is working on motion of the hand and arm. Because the paint reduces the friction between hand and paper, it is easier to get movement.

Painting with a brush can be a prewriting exercise for a client with hand injury. The brush handle can be built up with cylindrical foam padding for clients with arthritis, hand clients, or for those with weakened grip. Because watercolor requires little strength, it is an appropriate activity for someone who is very weak. Tempera and watercolor wash out of cloth easily and will not permanently stain bed clothes (Department of the Army, 1971).

Mental Health

Art techniques are most often used with psychiatric clients. These media allow for the most expression of feelings. Color, texture, patterns, and spacing can all be used to express the client's emotions. What the client says while working should be remembered and noted on the back of the artwork. This is frequently helpful to the psychiatrist and other staff members. Art offers many opportunities for clients to focus on problem areas. Working together in a room with other clients gives the client the opportunity to practice social skills.

Pediatrics

Drawing precedes writing as a way of expression. Young children start by making lines, then scribbles, circles with arms and legs and facial features, and then other shapes. Some feel that developmental maturation is easily visible in children's drawings. Thick kindergarten crayons are best for young children, as they have not developed enough fine motor control to work with regular crayons. With children, art is often the quickest way to see what is happening within them emotionally. They have not yet learned to censor their expression. The simplest materials—crayons, fingerpaint, or tempera paint with a brush—are often better than using complicated techniques. Young children need larger paper, 18 x 24 inches, as they have more difficulty with fine motor control. Manual dexterity can be improved with painting and drawing. The experience of art is usually so much fun for young children that they are seldom critical of the product.

Older children often enjoy the different techniques, such as crayon resist or crayon etching. Their hand control is usually adequate to accomplish the realism that children attempt in their art from ages 8 to 12 years. Colored pencils are often enjoyed by this age group (Harris, 1963; DiLeo, 1973; Gaitskell, Hurwitz, 1975).

Adolescents are usually self-conscious about their art. This can be minimized by doing abstract art, which allows them to avoid self-consciousness about their ability to draw realistically. They can enjoy patterns and new techniques that allow them to focus on the art rather than their drawing skill.

Because children's bodies are small, the amount of any toxic fume from permanent markers can be especially hazardous. Precautions must be taken with all such art materials to avoid toxic exposure (Anonymous, 1986).

Geriatrics

The first response that many older people give to requests that they participate in art activities is often, "I can't draw." Crafts that involve art such as toile painting or stencils may assist in easing older adults into art. It is important to use sophisticated adult materials like pen and ink rather than child-oriented materials like crayons. Playing classical music during the activity has been found to counteract older adults' feelings of being involved in a childish activity. Drawings and paintings offer older adults wonderful opportunities to reminisce. A therapist can help them focus on their own life by asking them to draw simple life experiences, or by asking them to draw simple things from their childhood or young adult life: food, tools, clothes, pets, and flowers. Many people are phobic about drawing human figures or faces. These could be incorporated into later sessions. Drawing memories provides an opportunity for older people to make peace with their life while they preserve it for others through pictures. Elders may want to share their artwork with grandchildren as a way of showing "this is how it was back then" (Drake, 1988).

CASE STUDY

Danny was a 42-year-old third-generation Japanese-American dock worker. While unloading a ship, his right arm was smashed and had to be amputated. He was right handed. He had an above-the-elbow amputation. This was a very traumatic event for Danny, as he had been earning his living by using his hands since he was 16 years old. His parents ran a small neighborhood grocery store, and Danny had worked in the store as far back as he could remember until he quit high school in his junior year. He took a job on his uncle's fishing boat. At age 22, in 1968, he joined the Navy. During his 4-year enlistment, he met men from all over the country. He worked on his GED (general education diploma) and completed it. It was his hope to attend college when he was discharged from service. When he got home, he had difficulty adjusting to shore life in the same way Vietnam veterans had trouble adapting to civilian life.

His childhood sweetheart got pregnant, so they got married. He took a job working on the docks. The union pay was good, though the work was hard and he had never envisioned himself as a laborer. Four children came within 8 years, and his view of himself as a man with responsibilities dimmed his youthful dreams.

The occupational therapist used the Model of Human Occupation. She visited Danny for the first time 5 days after the surgery. He was sitting on his bed just staring at the television set, which was showing a soap opera. It was obvious that he was not paying attention, just staring at the screen. He wore his pajama top over the bandaged stump so it was not immediately apparent which was the effected arm. Danny responded slowly and minimally to the therapist's introduction and explanation of the occupational therapy process he could expect. She asked Danny to remove his shirt and move his shoulder so she could see if he had any movement restriction. Though she could see that the stump was swollen even above the bandage, he appeared to have full range of motion. She unwrapped the stump to look at its condition. There was the normal redness where the flap was stitched. She checked his range of motion again and rewrapped the stump. They talked briefly about Danny's job because he assumed she would help him with employment. She explained her role in his total rehabilitation. Though she knew he had been told all this before, she also knew from a discussion of Danny's case at grand rounds that he was very depressed and confused. She knew that depressed people often forget what they have been told, so she felt it was a good idea to explain each team member's role again. She used the Assessment of Occupational Functioning screening instrument to guide her interview with him (Christiansen, Baum, 1991). She discussed the necessity of a program to learn one-handed skills. Danny's response was lukewarm.

The therapist wrote the following long-term treatment goals with Danny's tacit supervision:

*   To re-evaluate his own physical capacities and potential
*   To identify what matters most to him
*   To identify occupations/activities he enjoys
*   To examine the performance of roles most important to him
*   To develop the skills required for those roles

The next day, after range of motion exercises, she had Danny hold a pencil and write his name with his left hand. She began to ask him about his experiences in writing. He told of attending Japanese school in the Buddhist temple on Saturdays as a child. As they discussed this, he remembered having learned brush calligraphy. Sometimes the teacher had given lessons on sumi-e, Japanese ink painting. He had enjoyed that. They had sometimes carried the ink and brushes outside and painted objects in the temple garden. For a moment as they talked, it seemed he had forgotten his plight. The therapist took advantage of his more animated description and asked if he might like to try to do some ink painting again during his rehabilitation. His face fell as he looked where his right hand should have been. He just shook his head. The occupational therapist said, "Well, you need to begin to practice using that left hand. Let's try it." Danny looked crestfallen, but he didn't say no.

The therapist had to go to the Japanese variety store to purchase rice paper, bamboo brushes, and preground liquid sumi-e ink. The next day she carried these, along with a pair of left-handed scissors and the book, *The Living Art of Ink Painting*, by Ryozo Ogura (1968), into the room. Danny appeared as depressed as at the first visit, but she matter-of-factly put him through his exercises, his self-care training, and then assisted him in unrolling the rice paper, cutting off a piece, and opening the ink bottle. She directed him to paint his name with his left hand. He slowly picked up the brush and dipped it into the ink. As he applied the brush to the paper, it began to make a big spot where the brush touched. "I can't do this," he said. The occupational therapist reminded him that everything took practice. She left him trying his name for the third time.

The next day when she came back, he was sitting straighter. He showed her a piece of rice paper cut rather jaggedly with his name in English and Japanese calligraphy. He appeared proud of the work as he described his father's visit last evening and how his father had demonstrated what he could remember of calligraphy. They seemed to be able to talk about Japanese ink painting in a way they had been unable to share since Danny was a little boy. He said he thought he'd practice on it some more since that was what he always told his children about homework practice.

He was discharged and came to the outpatient clinic. His inpatient therapist was allowed to maintain him as her client in the outpatient clinic. His temporary prosthesis was not fine-tuned enough for him to attempt to paint with it. A few weeks later, however, when his permanent prosthesis had been fitted, the therapist began to work with him on using the bamboo sumi-e brush with his hook. She built up the handle so it was easier to grip. His first paintings were large figures, leaves, and fish because he was using gross shoulder motions (Figure 17-1). It was discouraging at first, as he felt he had no control. Often he also complained of phantom pain during the sessions. Gradually, his paintings began to show more refinement. Nonetheless, he began to prefer painting with his left hand rather than using the prosthesis.

The social worker worked with the Department of Vocational Rehabilitation and the union steward. They were able to get the shipping company that owned the dock where Danny worked to train him to do computer inventories of ship contents so he could return to full-time active employment rather than receiving disability money.

His renewed interest in Japanese calligraphy and art was shared by his family. As he became more skilled, one of his childhood friends who taught Japanese language in the Saturday Japanese school asked him to teach an occasional class on sumi-e. By this time he was able to grind his own ink and paint in a true traditional way, using both his right prosthesis and left hand.

DISCUSSION QUESTIONS

1. Cultural crafts can sometimes be used to motivate clients to attempt activities. What might be an appropriate cultural craft for an Italian? A Native American? A Central American? A Scandinavian?

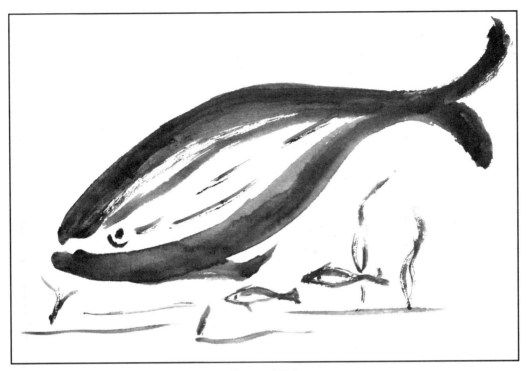

Figure 17-1.
Sumi-e painting of a fish.

2. If you were planning a session with a group mural, how would you assist clients in choosing a theme? How could you help them to avoid a situation in which everyone is allowed to work on any space they like, thus producing a fragmented effect?

3. In which other crafts you have studied so far could drawing and painting be used? How?

REFERENCES

Achterberg, J. (1985). *Imagery in healing.* Boston: New Science Library.

Androes, L., Dreyfus, E. A., & Bloesch, M. (1965). Diagnostic test battery for occupational therapy. *Am J Occup Ther, 19*(2), 53-59.

Anonymous. (1986). Hazards in arts & crafts. *Emergency Medicine. 18*(18), 60-64, 69, 73.

AOTA Practice Division. (1988). *Mental health information packet.* Rockville, MD: American Occupational Therapy Association.

Ascher, I. E. (1996). *Occupational therapy assessment tools: An annotated index* (2nd ed.). Bethesda, MD: American Occupational Therapy Association.

Betensky, M. (1973). *Self-discovery through self-expression.* Springfield, IL: Charles C. Thomas.

Buck, J. N. (1948). The house-tree-person techniques: a qualitative and quantitative scoring manual. *J Clin Psychol, 4,* 151-159.

Burns, R. C. & Kaufman, S. H. (1972). *Actions, styles and symbols in kinetic family drawings (K-F-D).* New York: Brunner/Mazel.

Christiansen, C., & Baum, C. (1991). *Occupational therapy: Overcoming human performance deficits.* Thorofare, NJ: SLACK Incorporated.

Department of the Army. (1971). *Craft techniques in occupational therapy.* Washington DC: U.S. Government Printing Office

Detre, K. C., et al. (1983). Roots of art therapy. *American Journal of Art Therapy, 20*(4), 111-123.

DiLeo, J. H. (1973). *Children's drawings as diagnostic aids.* New York: Brunner/Mazel.

Drake, L. M. (1988). Art media with aging adults: views from near the finish line. *Gerontology special interest section newsletter, 11*(3), 1-2.

Early, M. B. (1993). *Mental health concepts and techniques for the occupational therapy assistant.* New York: Raven Press.

Gaitskell, C. D., & Hurwitz, A. (1975). *Children and their art* (3rd ed.). New York: Harcourt, Brace, Jovanovitch.

Hammer, E. F. (1958). *The clinical application of projective drawings.* Springfield, IL: Charles C. Thomas.

Harris, D. B. (1963). *Children's drawings as measures of intellectual maturity.* New York: Harcourt, Brace and World, Inc.

Hemphill, B. J. (1982a). *The evaluative process in psychiatric occupational therapy.* Thorofare, NJ: SLACK Incorporated.

Hemphill, B. J. (1982b). *Training manual for the BH battery.* Thorofare, NJ: SLACK Incorporated.

Janson, A. (1995). *H. W. Janson's history of art* (5th ed.). New York: Harry N. Abrams, Inc.

Janson, H. W. (1969). *History of art* (2nd ed.). Englewood Cliffs, NJ: Prentice Hall.

Kaplan, H. I., & Sadock, B. J. (1981). *Modern synopsis of comprehensive textbook of psychiatry III* (3rd ed.). Baltimore: Williams & Wilkins.

Kaplan H. I., & Saddock, B. J. (1998). *Kaplan and Saddock's synopsis of psychiatry: Behavioral sciences/clinical psychiatry* (8th ed.). Baltimore: Williams & Wilkins.

Lewin, R. (1988). *In the age of mankind.* Washington DC: Smithsonian Books.

Liebman, M. (1986). *Art therapy for groups.* Cambridge, MA: Brookline Books.

Machover, K. (1949). *Personality projection in the drawing of the human figure.* Springfield, IL: Charles C. Thomas.

Ogura, R. (1968). *The lively art of ink painting.* Tokyo: Japan Publications.

Oster, G. D., & Gould, P. (1987). *Using drawings in assessment and therapy.* New York: Brunner/Mazel.

Rhyne, J. (1973). *The gestalt art experience.* Belmont,CA: Wadsworth Publishing Company, Inc.

Robbins, A. & Sibley, L. B. (1976). *Creative art therapy.* New York: Brunner/Mazel.

Siev, E., & Frieshtat, B. (1976). *Perceptual dysfunction in the adult stroke patient.* Thorofare, NJ: Charles B. Slack.

Ulman, E., & Dachinger, P. (eds.). (1975). *Art therapy in theory and practice.* New York: Schocken Books.

Urband, W. H. (1963). *The draw-a-person catalog for interpretive analysis.* Los Angeles: Western Psychological Services.

Wald, J. (1983). Alzheimer's disease and the role of art therapy in its treatment. *American Journal of Art Therapy, 22*(2), 57-64.

Willard, H. S., & Spackman, C. S. (1947). *Principles of occupational therapy.* Philadelphia: Lippincott.

OTHER FREQUENTLY USED CRAFTS

INTRODUCTION

Crafts become fads in a way similar to food and clothes. Photographs of occupational therapy in the 1920s and 1930s show basketry and working with straw (Howe, Schwartzberg, 1986). Books from the 1940s and 1950s show pictures of woodworking and looms for weaving and knotting (Colson, 1944; Department of the Army, 1951; Dunton, Licht, 1957; Haworth, MacDonald, 1946; Willard, Spackman, 1947). Books from the 1960s have more adaptive equipment and industrial or vocational pictures (Jones, 1969; MacDonald, 1960). By the 1970s, there were fewer craft photos, replaced by pictures of splints, pediatric developmental testing, and adaptive equipment (Jones, 1977; Hopkins, Smith, 1978; Willard, Spackman, 1971). This trend continued into the 1980s, with more pictures of vocational and work-hardening activities (Hopkins, Smith, 1983, 1988; Ryan, 1986). Photographs in occupational therapy books from the 1990s picture crafts as a historical artifact. In these books, even euphemisms for crafts such as *purposeful activity* have all but disappeared (Early, 1993; Christiansen, Baum, 1997; Neistadt, Crepeau, 1998; Sabonis-Chafee, Hussey, 1998). Within each of these decades, there have been other crafts that have held the limelight in occupational therapy clinics for brief spans of time. New crafts continue to be developed that fit current treatment situations such as decreased hospital stays and increasing numbers of elderly clients.

FREQUENCY OF USE

The term *minor media* is sometimes used to refer to crafts that receive less emphasis, while they may still be useful activities (Wilkinson, Heater, 1979). The orientation of the person defining the category will decide which media will be defined as minor. In this text it means those crafts that are used less frequently yet still have enough value to be something a therapist can use when necessary, even if they are not used often enough for the therapist to feel skilled in doing them. Crafts that could qualify as minor media are decoupage, stain frames, nature printing, and silk screening. Each of these crafts will be discussed briefly.

INDIVIDUAL MINOR MEDIA

Decoupage

This craft has a French name. Couper, the root word in decoupage, means to cut. Some craft historians claim the craft developed in France and some say Italy. Decoupage was originally intended to be an inexpensive way of reproducing the look of oriental lacquerware. Pictures were cut out and glued to lacquered objects, then covered with clear lacquer to simulate the handpainted designs on oriental furniture. It quickly spread to other countries as a decorative technique.

Though the original method took a great deal of time to complete, modern products have made it a simple and satisfying craft for clients. New one-coat finishes have been developed to simulate those that formerly required 10 coats of varnish or lacquer (Bodger, Brock, 1976; Reader's Digest, 1979; VanZandt, 1973). Decoupage can be applied to glass, porcelain, or wood. The techniques for wood are described below.

SUPPLIES
- Wooden decoupage plaque
- Fine sandpaper
- Wood stain
- Decoupage finish
- Pictures from greeting cards or pictures printed on other thick paper
- Scissors
- Small glue brush
- Finish brush with 2 1/2-inch bristles
- Cup to hold decoupage finish
- Brayer or rolling pin

PROCESS
1. Sand the wooden plaque.
2. Wipe on the wood stain and allow it to dry.

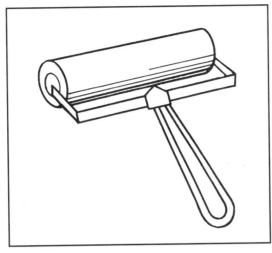

Figure 18-1.
Brayer.

3. Cut out a picture and try it on the plaque for correct placement.
4. If the edges are thick, thin them by sanding gently from the back so they will be flat.
5. With a small brush, apply the decoupage finish, which works as glue, to the back of the picture.
6. Place the picture, glue side down, on the plaque.
7. With the rolling pin or brayer (Figure 18-1), gently roll out any bubbles under the picture. Allow this to dry.
8. Apply a coat of decoupage finish to the picture and wood, and allow it to dry.

Perhaps the best thing about decoupage is that a very nice product can be produced so simply. It allows a client with very diminished function to make a nice object. Most decoupage finish is neither flammable nor toxic, so it is not a hazard for low-functioning clients. It can be used to preserve personally valuable mementos like graduation or birth announcements. The one drawback for the modern short-stay clinic is the series of waiting periods while glue or finish dries. The client may leave before the finish is completely dry. Though this craft is less used than it was in the 1970s, it is a traditional method that will continue to be useful.

Stain Frames

Stain frames are fairly new compared to other crafts in this text. It is a short-term structured process using preformed plastic (styrene) forms. Glass stain paints are applied to the areas between the raised outline ridges. The finished product simulates stained glass. They can be used as suncatchers or holiday ornaments. Permanent markers or acrylic paints can be used for an opaque effect.

Stain frames are a simple one-step activity: simply applying the colors to the frame. Cleaning up and putting a hanger in the ring at the top completes this project. Because of its simplicity, it is well-adapted to modern-day clinics in which clients often have a time-limited session and tend to be sicker at the time they are treated than they were in the past when hospital stays were longer. In some ways, stain frames are like paint-by-number in that the client is not challenged by too many decisions.

Stain frames are appropriate for clients working on fine coordination/dexterity and motor control. Because stain frames are unbreakable, they can be used with clients who have grip or balance problems and tend to drop objects.

Nature Printing

This is another craft in which an extremely simple four-step process produces an interesting and clear design. Six x 9-inch sun-sensitive paper with objects on it is exposed to the sun. Wherever the object blocks out the sun, the paper is white. Areas exposed to the sun become bright blue. The only materials needed are the nature print paper, objects for the design, and tap water.

PROCESS

1. Arrange the objects on the paper. Possible objects could be keys, leaves, cut paper designs, buttons, lace, or crochet doilies.
2. Put the paper with objects in place in the sun for 15 minutes.
3. Remove the objects and immerse the paper in tap water.
4. Spread the wet paper on newspaper to dry. To keep the wet paper from curling, tack each corner down to cardboard with straight pins.

Almost any client will enjoy this rather magical craft process; however, as a therapeutic media, it is probably most appropriate for clients who have poor attention spans and need quick gratification. Clients on sun-sensitive medication such as Thorazine and some antibiotics need to be cautioned about the hazards of staying out in the sun with their design. The nature print makes a nice design for the front of a greeting card or to decoupage.

Printing

The first printing was developed in China in approximately 200 A.D. These first prints were what we today call monoprints, or simple prints. A design is made with ink, and another paper is pressed on the ink to make a mirror image. Then it was discovered that stone carvings or seal rings could be used to print. The surface of the carving was rubbed with ink and then paper was pressed on the ink. A simple carved design could be used over and over. In about 600 A.D., the Chinese invented the process for woodblock printing in which a design was carved into a flat woodblock. The block was covered with ink by a brayer or roller (see

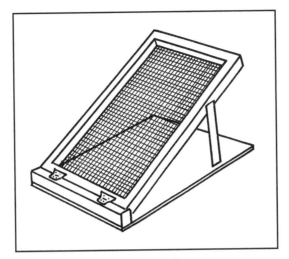

Figure 18-2.
Silk screen frame.

Figure 18-1) and then pressed onto the paper. The first European wood-block prints appeared in the 1400s. Metal etchings developed later in that same century. Lithography printing using flat stones with an ink-absorbent design was created in the late 1700s.

Silk-screen on cloth, sometimes called serigraphy, was developed in the first decade of this century in England. This makes it a comparative-ly modern craft. It is a more complex process of printing in which ink is pushed onto paper or cloth through a stencil design fixed on tightly stretched fine fabric mesh. T-shirts are commonly decorated this way. Its complexity may be the reason it is so rarely used (*Reader's Digest,* 1979; Hobson, 1970; Kent, Cooper, 1966).

Typesetting and printing presses have often been used in occupation-al therapy (Department of the Army, 1951, 1971; Dunton, Licht, 1957; Jones, 1977; Office of the Surgeon General, 1945). Printing presses are almost never found in clinics today. Few commercial establishments have typesetting anymore. They use photo typesetting. The demise of the print-ing press in occupational therapy clinics parallels its demise in commer-cial print shops. Artists may be the main users of actual printing press-es for the processes of etching and lithography.

Silk-screen

Silk-screen designs can be blocked out by brushing glue, lacquer, lith-ographer's tushe, or shellac right onto the screen. A lithographer's cray-on can be used to draw on the cloth, or a special silk-screen film can be affixed to the mesh. A simple way to achieve a silk-screen effect is the paper stencil method. Materials needed for this process are:
- Silk-screen box with mesh attached (Figure 18-2)
- Paper
- Acrylic or water-soluble printer's ink

- Squeegee
- Scissors

PROCESS

1. Cover the work area with newspapers.
2. Place the paper on which the print will be made on the newspaper.
3. Cut a paper design and position it under the silk-screen on top of the paper to be printed.
4. Squeeze ink onto the screen and use the squeegee to push the ink through the cloth and onto the design and bottom paper. Do not thin the ink. Thicker ink produces a clearer design.
5. When the screen is lifted, the cut design will adhere to the silk. Remove the printed paper below and replace with a clean sheet.
6. Repeat steps 4 and 5 until the desired number of prints are made.
7. Remove the paper design and discard it. Immediately wash the screen and squeegee with soap and water.

This method produces only simple, one-color designs. A thin paper used to make the cut design will result in a thin coat of ink on the printed paper. Thick paper used to make the design allows a thick layer of ink on the printed paper. Tracing paper or other nonabsorbent paper is not good for the cut design, as it will not adhere to the mesh to allow for more than one print. Physically, this method requires good upper extremity strength and coordination, prehension, and grasp (Kent, Cooper, 1966; Hamill, Oliver, 1989).

Linoleum Prints

The techniques for linoleum block and woodblock printing are basically the same. A design is cut into the top of the block, inked, and printed. The picture is inverted in this printing process, so all words or lettering must be carved backward.

SUPPLIES
- Block with at least 1/8-inch thick linoleum
- Carbon paper
- Linoleum lino cutters or wood-carving tools
- Brayer (see Figure 18-1)
- 8 x 11-inch glass or lucite window pane
- Water-soluble printer's ink
- 8 1/2 x 11-inch drawing paper or manila paper
- Newspapers
- Bracer board (see Figure 7-10)
- Paper towels

PROCESS

1. Cover the work area with newspaper.
2. Reproduce the desired design on the linoleum surface using carbon paper.
3. Cut the outline of the design into the linoleum with a lino cutter, which has a small blade in a loop shape on the end of the handle.
4. Gouge out the design where desired using a gouge with the block braced against a bracer board for support and safety.
5. Run a proof on a paper towel.
   a. Roll ink over the glass pane with the brayer.
   b. Roll the inked brayer over the linoleum surface.
   c. Press the linoleum onto the paper towel on a pad of newspapers.
6. If the proof is acceptable, continue printing on the drawing paper.
7. If the proof is unacceptable, wash off the ink. Dry the block and continue carving out the linoleum and printing until a satisfactory proof is run.
8. Wash the block, brayer, and inking pane with soap and water (*Reader's Digest*, 1979; Kent, Cooper, 1966).

Linoleum printing takes good upper extremity strength and control. Cutting the linoleum requires good hand strength and fine motor coordination. Use of the brayer elicits elbow flexion and extension. Some clients may substitute trunk motion for arm motion and should be observed and guided to achieve the desired movement (Hamill, Oliver, 1989). Depressed or suicidal clients will require the usual precautions with sharp tools. Teenagers may enjoy these techniques, but they are probably too difficult for children younger than 8 or 9 years of age.

Innertube Printing

This method of printing is similar to linoleum and woodblock printing during the actual printing process. However, the process of making the design to be printed is much easier. A design is drawn on a used tire innertube. The design is cut out with regular craft scissors. The design pieces are arranged as desired on the woodblock background and glued in place with water-resistant glue. After the glue is dry, the linoleum printing process from step 5 onward is followed. Because this process uses fewer and less dangerous tools, it can be used by children and lower-functioning clients. Because it is easier, it is also quicker and more adaptable for today's short hospital stays. All of these methods—wood, linoleum, and innertube block printing—produce attractive greeting cards and stationery.

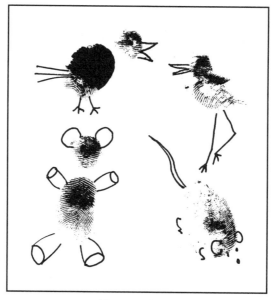

Figure 18-3.
Fingerprint designs.

Vegetable Prints

Vegetable prints make interesting repetitive designs for gift-wrap, book covers, or cloth.

SUPPLIES

- Raw carrots, potatoes, turnips, or other solid vegetables
- Paring knife
- Potato peeler
- Ink stamp pad and ink
- Paper towels
- Paper or fabric to be printed
- Newspapers

PROCESS

1. Cover the work area with newspaper.
2. Cross-cut the vegetable so there is a flat surface for carving the design.
3. Trace a simple shaped design like a triangle, square, star, or four-petal flower on the flat surface with the tip of the knife or a pen.
4. Incise the outline to 1/4-inch deep. This makes it easier to cut away or gouge out the background. The potato peeler tip may be useful for carving out corners of the design.
5. Press the cut surface onto the inked stamp pad and print a proof on a paper towel.
6. If the proof is satisfactory, proceed to print the design on paper or cloth.
7. Clean up.

Because of the inexpensiveness and availability of the materials and tools, this is popular for all ages. The same upper extremity strength and coordination requirements and suicidal precautions of other printing apply to vegetable printing.

Fingerprint Design

Another kind of printing for all age groups is fingerprint designs. Simply press a finger or thumb on an inked stamp pad, then press it on paper. When the print is dry, embellish it with arms, legs, or other features to make an entertaining, easy design that requires almost no strength (Figure 18-3).

There are many other minor crafts that therapists can use to offer variety and richness to their activity choices in working with clients. Craft materials manufacturers continue to develop new ideas for projects to make in the clinic. A visit to craft vendor booths at conferences is an opportunity to learn about these new materials and projects.

REFERENCES

Bodger, L., & Brock, D. (1976). *The crafts engagement calendar 1976.* New York: Universe Books.

Christiansen, C., & Baum, C. (1997), *Occupational therapy: Enabling function and well-being* (2nd ed.). Thorofare, NJ: SLACK Incorporated.

Colson, J. H. C, (1944). *The rehabilitation of the injured: Occupational therapy.* London: Cassell and Company.

Department of the Army. (1951). *Occupational therapy.* Washington DC: U.S. Government Printing Office.

Department of the Army. (1971). *Craft techniques in occupational therapy.* Washington DC: U.S. Government Printing Office.

Dunton, W. R., & Licht, S. (1957). *Occupational therapy principles and practice.* Springfield, IL: Charles C. Thomas.

Early, M. B. (1993), *Mental health concepts and techniques for the occupational therapy assistant.* New York: Raven Press.

Hamill, C. M., & Oliver, R. C. (1989). *Therapeutic activity for the handicapped elderly.* Gaithersburg. MD: Aspen Publishers.

Haworth, N. A., & MacDonald, E. M. (1946). *Theory of occupational therapy.* Baltimore: Williams & Wilkins

Hobson, J. (1970). *Dyed and printed fabrics.* Wood Ridge, NJ: the Dryad Press.

Hopkins, H. L., & Smith, H. D. (1978). *Willard and Spackman's occupational therapy* (5th ed.). Philadelphia: Lippincott.

Hopkins, H. L., & Smith, H. D. (1983). *Willard and Spackman's occupational therapy* (6th ed.). Philadelphia: Lippincott.

Hopkins, H. L., & Smith, H. D. (1988). *Willard and Spackman's occupational therapy* (7th ed.). Philadelphia: Lippincott.

Howe, M., & Schwartzberg, S. (1986). *A functional approach to group work in occupational therapy.* Philadelphia: Lippincott.

Jones, M. S. (1969). *An approach to occupational therapy.* London: Butterworth.

Jones, M. S. (1977). *An approach to occupational therapy.* London: Butterworth.

Kent, C., & Cooper, M. (1966). *Simple printmaking.* New York: Watson-Gauptill Publications.

MacDonald, E. M. (ed.). (1960). *Occupational therapy in rehabilitation.* Baltimore: Williams & Wilkins.

Neistadt, M. E., & Crepeau, E. B. (1998). *Willard and Spackman's occupational therapy* (9th ed.). Philadelphia: Lippincott.

Office of the Surgeon General. (1945). *Curing by printing: Printing activities in occupational therapy.* New York: American Type Founders.

Reader's Digest. (1979). *Crafts and hobbies.* Pleasantville, NY: Reader's Digest Association, Inc.

Ryan, S. (ed.). (1986). *The certified occupational therapy assistant: Roles and responsibilities.* Thorofare, NJ: SLACK Incorporated.

Sabonis-Chafee, B., & Hussey, S. M. (1998). *Introduction to occupational therapy* (2nd ed.). St. Louis: Mosby.

VanZandt, E. (1973). *Crafts for fun and profit.* London: Aldus Books.

Wilkinson, V. C., & Heater, S. L. (1979). *Therapeutic media and techniques of application: A guide for aActivities therapists.* New York: Van Nostrand Reinhold Company.

Willard, H. S., & Spackman, C. S. (1947). *Principles of occupational therapy.* Philadelphia: Lippincott.

Willard, H. S., & Spackman, C. S. (1971). *Occupational therapy* (4th ed.). Philadelphia: Lippincott.

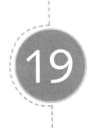

CRAFTS FROM FOUND MATERIALS FOR HOME HEALTH PRACTICE

INTRODUCTION

While occupational therapists have been involved in home health for more than 25 years, this field of practice has only burgeoned in the last decade, as hospital stays have shortened and sicker clients have gone home (Levine, Corcoran, Gitlin, 1993; Joe, 1996). As the health care system has become more streamlined and cost conscious, the emphasis has focused on functional limitations and how they are documented. The therapist's role as a teacher is more important than as a provider of treatment (Levine, Corcoran, Gitlin, 1993; Atchison, 1997; McGuire, 1997; Stahl, 1998). The same core values of occupational therapy apply in the home as in the hospital (Opacich, 1997). Since the "bottom line" or "cost containment" is at the center of practice today, one way to contain costs is to use found art and craft materials rather than expensive commercial materials. Found materials are anything that was not intentionally prepared to be used to make crafts. Creative therapists have always used what others see as "throw-aways." In the past, it was common for a therapist to receive a stack of something such as medication cups and think, "Hmmm, now what can I do with those? Maybe two cups can be put rim to rim to make holiday decorations." The current medical climate makes this process of recycling a necessity (Breines, 1998; Ehrlich, Piersol, 1997). When the price of a simple craft kit can start at $3.00, its cost is a consideration in planning treatment. Found materials are especially convenient in home health because it is impossible for a therapist to carry a full spectrum of possible crafts in her car. A box with some basic craft tools and supplies, such as those listed below, can allow the therapist to improvise on-the- spot from found art and craft materials that are usually present in every household (Adams, 1989; 1991a; 1991b).

Tools and Supplies to Make Most Found Crafts

- Kitchen scissors
- Pliers
- White glue
- Super glue
- Glue gun
- Spray adhesive
- Pressing iron
- Hammer
- Sponge
- Brushes
- Water-based paints
- Toothpicks (Stribling, 1970)

Categories of Found Materials

HOUSEHOLD ITEMS

- Plastic lids
- Empty milk or juice containers
- Cardboard toilet paper rolls
- Plastic sewing thread spools
- Egg cartons
- Styrofoam trays from meat, cookies, etc.
- Empty glass jars with lids
- Aluminum pie tins
- Tin cans
- Oatmeal boxes
- Strawberry baskets
- Flower pots (plastic and clay)
- Popsicle sticks
- Flour and salt

NATURAL MATERIALS

- Driftwood
- Twigs
- Leaves
- Grasses
- Shells
- Feathers

- Bones
- Stones
- Gourds
- Pinecones

HARDWARE ITEMS

- Old keys
- Sparkplugs
- Springs
- Nails
- Hinges
- Lengths of chain
- Wire
- PVC pipe

SCRAP PAPER

- Discarded wrapping paper
- Old magazines
- Greeting cards
- Wallpaper sample books
- Newspaper
- Brown paper bags
- Newspaper used for cushioning in packing boxes

FIBER AND FABRIC

- String
- Yarn
- Gift ribbon
- Old socks
- Fabric scraps
- Embroidery floss
- Discarded clothing
- Old curtains
- Ragged dishtowels

Possible Projects to Make with Found Materials

- Masks
- Greeting cards
- Posters
- Collages
- Montages
- Window decorations
- Sculptures
- Mobiles

- Wall hangings
- Decorated containers
- Puppets
- Gifts

A therapist can ask a client to choose from the mentioned list of possible projects to make and then assist the client in finding the materials to make the project in his or her home. The client's culture will determine what possible craft ingredients will be found. Culture is a most important element in home-health occupational therapy (Piersol, 1998; Weinstein, 1997).

Native Americans were especially good at utilizing natural materials. Children often enjoy making Native American objects and clothing. This process allows them to learn about Native American culture as well as gain respect for natural materials such as pine cones, feathers, and shells (Carlson, 1994; Leftwich, 1970). An example of how one discard can be made into three different craft projects illustrates the versatility of found material crafts. An aluminum soup can can be made into a candle holder, pencil holder, or wishing well.

Aluminum Can Candle Holder

MATERIALS
- Aluminum soup can
- Water
- Hammer
- Nail
- Paper
- Pencil
- Tape
- Votive candle

PROCESS
1. Wash the can out.
2. Fill the can with water.
3. Put it in the freezer over night.
4. Draw a design on a piece of paper to fit around the can.
5. Remove the can from the freezer.
6. Tape the drawing to the can.
7. Place the can on a pad of towels to keep it from rolling.
8. Use a hammer and nail to make a small hole every 1/4 to 1/2 inch along the lines of the drawing.
9. Put the can in the sink to allow the ice to thaw.

10. Let the can dry (drying the inside can be hazardous, as the rough edges of the aluminum holes can scratch skin).
11. Put a votive candle in the bottom and light it.
12. This makes an attractive candle holder that is simple to make. The candlelight shows through the pattern of holes.

Aluminum Can Pencil Holder

MATERIALS

- Aluminum soup can
- Yarn scraps
- White glue
- Tape
- Scissors
- Glue brush

PROCESS

1. Wash out and dry the aluminum soup can.
2. Use scraps of yarn to wind around the can, starting at the bottom.
3. Tape the end of the yarn to the bottom of the soup can.
4. Place a horizontal line of glue on the can starting where the yarn passes from under the bottom of the can and begin to wind the yarn over and into the glue.
5. Continue this process until the yarn reaches the top rim of the can.
6. Snip off the yarn and firmly glue the end.
7. Allow the yarn to dry several hours.
8. Brush a layer of white glue over the yarn and allow it to dry.
9. This makes a colorful project that even children can do. Using variegated colored yarn makes an especially interesting pencil holder.

Aluminum Can Wishing Well Flower Container

MATERIALS

- Aluminum soup can
- Glue gun and glue
- Small stones of two different colors

PROCESS

1. Wash the aluminum can inside and out.
2. Completely dry the can.
3. Make a drainage hole in the bottom of the can with a hammer and nail.
4. Gather small smooth stones of two different colors.

5. Wash the stones and allow them to dry.
6. Sort the stones into two colors.
7. Heat the glue gun with glue stick inside.
8. Starting at the bottom of the side of the soup can, apply a large drop of glue.
9. Quickly stick a stone into the glue.
10. Continue this process until the outside of the can is covered in stones, except for the top row.
11. Glue the second color of stones around the top.
12. Fill with dirt and add a small plant.

These examples show the variety of projects that can be made from the same found materials. The concept of found materials also fits with the idea of helping our environment by recycling. This is an idea to encourage with all client populations.

CASE STUDY

Agnes, an 82-year-old Caucasian retired psychiatric nurse, is receiving home health occupational therapy for her Colles' fracture of the wrist, which occurred during a burglary. Agnes still lives in the home she shared with her husband while they raised their three children. The houses in her neighborhood had all been built as a development during the 1950s. Her husband died 15 years ago. Agnes remained in her home in a neighborhood where she knew everyone within a three-block area. Gradually, the neighborhood began to change. As the neighbors her age began to move into assisted living residences or died, their homes were resold at prices that were considered low cost. The house on the corner became a crack house. Other houses were gradually allowed to run down. Agnes had felt safe until a crack-cocaine addict broke into her house during one late afternoon. She had heard the loud noise of the burglar breaking in the back door of the sunroom. She struggled up out of the rocking chair where she was dozing. He physically attacked her when she met him near the door between the sunroom and the kitchen. He knocked her down and she broke her wrist as she attempted to break her fall onto the kitchen floor. The burglar hit her several times so that she had several large bruises and a black eye. He took her purse, which was laying by the telephone in the kitchen, and ran out the backdoor because he heard the postman put the mail through the front door mail-slot. Agnes called out to the postman, who ran to the neighbor's house and called the police. She spent several days in the hospital for evaluation and treatment.

The agency providing home health care was part of a total hospital plan of a preferred provider organization. The hospital also has a Level II occupational therapy fieldwork program. Students in the occupational therapy internship spend the last month accompanying clinical faculty on morning home health rounds and working with hospitalized clients in the afternoon. The occupational therapist had seen Agnes twice before she was discharged.

Her wrist was immobilized in a cast, but her fingers were free. In addition to a simple sensory test of Agnes' fingers to make sure there was no loss of sensation, the occupational therapist administered the Assessment of Occupational Functioning (AOF) (Christiansen, Baum, 1991). The Model of Human Occupation was the underlying theory in the occupational therapy department. The OTR (occupational therapist, registered) learned that Agnes enjoyed many crafts, talking on the telephone with her friends, attending church, and visiting with neighborhood children. However, she felt that she had lost control of a good part of her life when she thought about her vulnerability to the burglar. Agnes demonstrated some symptoms of post-traumatic stress disorder (APA, 1994). She experienced flashbacks whenever someone knocked on her hospital door. She demonstrated an exaggerated startle response and would begin to tremble and cower. When the OTR tried to get her to retell what she had experienced, Agnes was unable to recall what happened after she saw the burglar. The OTR decided to complete the assessment when she visited Agnes at home, as she felt the questions would be more realistically dealt with in her natural home environment. Additionally, she would be able to perform a self-care assessment in the client's home. Because of her post-traumatic stress disorder symptoms, her physician referred her to psychiatry while she was still hospitalized. The psychiatrist made a follow-up appointment for her to visit him in his office 2 weeks after discharge.

Agnes' daughter from New Orleans took a week of leave from her job to be with her mother during her first days at home. During that week, the occupational therapist made her first visit. The second visit, the fieldwork student accompanied her. They sat in the breakfast area of the kitchen to complete the assessment and plan Agnes's treatment. The OTR encouraged the student to complete the AOF. A window sill full of African violets with many dead leaves showed that the plants had not had care during her hospital stay. The coffee table, visible through the kitchen door, was covered with new potted plants Agnes had received in the hospital. Though dusty, her home did not contain the stacks of memorabilia, tables full of medication containers, and old publications found in the homes of many elderly.

The student was able to get Agnes to tell about how last year she was involved in the garden club project in which they made dried flower bouquets to sell at the community festival in the park. She had cut and dried flowers from her own garden. Agnes was unable to think of any goals she had for her future. When she began to think about the future, she knew her friends would want her to move into the retirement residence, but she felt unable to think of moving. She felt able to do most things she needed to do for herself each day except bathe. The cast on her arm prevented her from taking a shower. The home health nurse had shown her how to put a plastic bag over the cast, but she had been unable to do it as she felt insecure in getting in the shower. The occupational therapist and student evaluated her home for safety hazards (Piersol, 1998; Collins, Beissner, Krout, 1998).

She missed being able to work in her flower garden. She thought she might be able to hoe with one hand but hadn't felt able to get out and try yet. She also missed her grandchildren, who all live in other cities. She has allowed the visits of neighborhood children to substitute for the missing grandchildren. She would often help these substitute grandchildren in doing projects. This gave the fieldwork student the idea of how she might be able to utilize found craft materials to assist Agnes in continuing to do projects with the children. Agnes lives on a fixed income of her husband's pension and her own social security, she was not able to afford many extra expenses. She was unable to hold traditional American scissors because of her cast, so the fieldwork student began to have her experiment with craft snips and squeezer-type scissors on a variety of materials. The fieldwork student went to the kitchen with Agnes and found plastic sheets that come under cream cheese, which Agnes always washed and saved, and thin cardboard from a cereal box to practice cutting on. While getting these materials, the fieldwork student discovered that one cupboard was full of clean styrofoam trays, empty glass, plastic jars, aluminum pie tins, etc. Agnes explained she had always saved such things since the Depression in the 1930s.

At the end of the session, the student discussed what goals Agnes thought she should have. Her first goal was to recover the full use of her hand and arm when her fracture healed. Complete self-care was her long-term goal. She then thought she ought to have a goal of doing something each day with the neighbor children so she would not be lonely, as she was confined to the house unless someone from her church came to take her shopping or to church. To insure her safety from further burglary or violence, she wanted to have wrought iron safety doors installed for both the front and back exits. This would allow her to stay in her house with peace of mind.

The third occupational therapy home health visit was the last, since the preferred provider organization (PPO) case manager determined that Agnes could get the most benefit by outpatient visits for upper extremity strengthening when her cast came off and visits to the counselor in the psychiatrist's office for the post-traumatic stress disorder. So the fieldwork student and occupational therapist spent a good amount of time planning how they could most efficiently use the 45 minutes allowed for this last home visit to teach Agnes whatever she needed to know for managing her life in her house and community. Her performance of activities of daily living was independent except for the bath help she received from the nursing assistant. Her social behavior was the thing with which occupational therapy could provide the most help. They planned to have Agnes make a list of places where she could assist children with crafts on a regular basis, rather than trusting the haphazard visits of the neighborhood children. Then they planned to assist her to find the correct phone numbers so she could contact these places. They anticipated that she would name the school, Sunday school, and local community center recreation program. They expected to assist her to get in contact with the transportation service of the area Agency on Aging.

DISCUSSION QUESTIONS

1. Are there any found crafts Agnes could use to sublimate her anger at being burglarized?
2. How can the therapist and student document what they do with Agnes so that the notes show how important it is for her to be able to do the crafts she does with children?
3. In a multi-cultural community, what differences might be expected in relation to what found materials might be in the homes of various ethnic groups?

REFERENCES

Adams, G. (1989). *How to make craft recipes.* Green Oaks, IL: Oak Springs Publications.

Adams, G. (1991a). *How to make craft projects From Nature.* Libertyville, IL: Oak Springs Publications.

Adams, G. (1991b). *How to make craft projects from recycled materials,* Libertyville, IL: Oak Springs Publications

American Psychiatric Association. (1994). *Diagnostic and statistical manual of mental disorders* (4th ed.). Washington DC: American Psychiatric Association

Atchison, B. (1997). Occupational therapy in home health: Rapid changes need proactive planning. *Am J Occup Ther, 51*(6), 406-409.

Breines, E. (1998). The case for recycling "stuff." *Advance for Occupational Therapy Practitioners, 14*(24), 5.

Carlson, L. (1994). *More than moccasins: A kid's activity guide to traditional North American indian life.* Chicago: Chicago Review Press.

Christiansen, C., & Baum, C. (1991). *Occupational therapy: Overcoming human performance deficits.* Thorofare, NJ: SLACK Incorporated.

Collins, J., Beissner, K. L,. & Krout, J. A. (1998). Home health physical therapy; Practice patterns in western New York. *Phys Ther, 78*(2), 170-179.

Ehrlich, P., & Piersol, C. (1997). How you can succeed as a home care therapist, *Advance for Occupational Therapists, 13*(43), 12.

Joe, B. E. (1996). Homecare; growth and change. *OT Week, 10*(45), 14-15.

Leftwich, R. L. (1970). *Arts and crafts of the Cherokee.* Cherokee, NC: Cherokee Publications.

Levine, R. E., Corcoran, M. A., & Gitlin, L. N. (1993). Home care and private practice. In: H. L. Hopkins & H. D. Smith (eds.). *Willard and Spackman's occupational therapy* (8th ed.). Philadelphia: Lippincott.

McGuire, M. J. (1997). Documenting progress in home care. *Am J Occup Ther, 51*(6), 436-445.

Opacich, K. J. (1997). Moral tensions and obligations of occupational therapy practitioners providing home care. *Am J Occup Ther, 51*(6), 430-435.

Piersol, C. V. (1998). How is OT in the home unique? *Advance for Occupational Therapists, 14*(8):7.

Stahl, C. (1998). Putting pediatric home care in better focus. *Advance for Occupational Therapists, 1*(14), 32-33.

Stribling, M. L. (1970). *Art from found materials.* New York: Crown Publishers.

Weinstein, M. (1997). Bringing family-centered practices into home health. *OT Practice, 2*(7), 35-38.

MISCELLANEOUS
CREATIVE MEDIA

INTRODUCTION

While we usually do not think of performance activities as crafts, it is common in theater work to speak of the acting craft. A craft is also defined as an activity that is done skillfully and ingeniously (*Webster's New Collegiate Dictionary*, 1969). This definition is used in this chapter to explain the inclusion of face painting, clowning, pantomime, and magic. Face painting, clowning, and miming—each an individual craft with its own merit—fit together. Faces are painted before both clowning and miming. Clowns wear make-up and also include pantomime in their acts. Most pantomime artists paint their faces and appear clownish. The three are often an integral part of a whole act. Noncompetitive games are also mentioned in this chapter as creative treatment media.

FACE PAINTING

This creative medium is often done at craft fairs and festivals where clowns and mime artists are also seen. Make-up for actors and clowns has been around for centuries. Face painting is a direct descendent of clown make-up and can be done with cosmetic face make-up. However, it is more permanent and gives a professional look if done with grease paint or theatrical make-up. Cosmetic make-up is more likely to run and smear. Grease paint will last longer and tolerate more wear and tear.

Supplies

- Paper and pencil
- Grease paint
- Make-up brushes
- Baby oil
- Talcum powder
- Facial tissue

Process

1. It is best to draw a face with a plan in mind for the make-up (Figure 19-1).
2. Brushes are used to apply face paint or grease paint. Apply colors in this order: white, pastels, primary colors, then black.
3. Powder each color after applying it. Brush excess powder away with a powder brush.
4. Clean grease paint from brushes with baby oil. Wipe the brushes dry.
5. Disinfect the brushes between clients.
6. Check face paint in the mirror.

The main precautions for using face paint are to be aware of allergies to make-up and avoid breathing the talcum powder. Face painting should be avoided by respiratory clients or those with dermatitis or acne.

Children and teenagers especially enjoy face painting. Face painting is almost a prerequisite for clowning and mime. In both of these crafts, most of the face is usually painted. Often for children and teens, just a flower, teardrop, or leaf design is sufficient rather than painting the whole face (Baygan, 1982; Buchman, 1975; Harris, 1985; Stolzenberg, 1981).

CLOWNING

Almost every culture has some form of clown character. Clowning is a kind of acting in which the actor wears stylized make-up and a costume. There is a cartoonlike quality to a clown act. Clowns help us laugh at our own human foibles and inadequacies. Clowning offers clients the opportunity to act silly in an acceptable caricature of themselves or others (Harris, 1985; Stolzenberg, 1981; Harzberg, Moss, 1924).

Clowning takes thought and planning, which are areas of frequent therapeutic focus in cognition and goal setting. Clients must think through the effect that they wish to achieve, then plan how they can accomplish that effect. There are opportunities to work in pairs or groups, as most clown acts involve team work. Generally, the client will have to be functioning well enough to appreciate humorous situations. The severely depressed, schizophrenic, and mentally retarded clients may

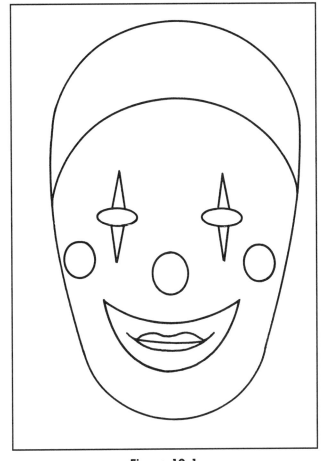

Figure 19-1.
Make-up face plan.

have difficulty organizing and carrying out comedy scenarios, while they may enjoy watching others perform clowning. Some clients with personality disorders could use this medium to exaggerate their aberrant responses to situations and people. Imagine a borderline personality-disordered client clutching at someone and screeching, "Don't leave me alone. I can't stand it." Alcoholics and drug abusers may enjoy playing the drunk. This process can help them develop insight into society's reaction to them.

For the physically disabled, playing the comical side of a disability can offer an emotional outlet for feelings about their situation. There has been an effort to use comedy to increase public awareness of disabilities. Comedy and clowning are seen as ways to alter the public's attitude about this sensitive subject (Milner, 1987a).

MIME

Mime and pantomime are used interchangeably here, as one term is just an abbreviation of the other. Gesture and pose, which are the bases of pantomime, were probably the first human means of communication. They are the most universal forms of communication. When communicating with someone who speaks a foreign language, we liberally augment speech with gestures.

Pantomime basically means storytelling through bodily movements and facial expression. Some attribute its development to the Greeks who so richly developed drama and its associated techniques, such as mime. Others say earliest humans mimicked animal movements as part of storytelling and worship. Tribal dances of Native Americans, Arabs, and Africans are indeed pantomime dances. They often do a pantomime of the hunt as preparation for actually going to hunt. Most European and British people have developed forms of pantomime. Charlie Chaplin may be the best mime artist America produced. Acting is native to humans and comes before speaking in the same way drawing comes before writing. Occupational therapists have been using drama techniques for many decades (Phillips, 1996; Keysell, 1975; Pardoe, 1931).

The main purpose in using mime with clients is to help them learn to communicate better and understand the body language of others. Second, pantomime is for fun. Third, it may be used to enact or reenact a client's problem situation. Start each mime session with a warm-up. In warming up, the clients can stretch, explore their body movements by keeping all but one part fixed, or by anchoring one part and moving all the others (Phillips, 1996). Music or rhythm instruments can be used to stimulate movement. An appropriate warm-up for children ages 3 to 8 years could be pretending to be a wind-up toy. The therapist would demonstrate with a real wind-up toy, then pretend to wind the child up. Other warm-ups for children could be pantomimes of different kinds of balls, animals, or vehicles. Warm-ups for children ages 8 to 12 years could be occupational or sports related, such as shooting a basketball. Teenagers may relate more to romantic dramatization or putting on make-up and clothes for warm-ups. This allows clients to get into the mood. Adults can be asked to do movements that simulate openness or closedness, nearness or distance. Such options allow adult clients to use just a hand if they are inhibited about body movement or to use the whole body if they feel less self-conscious. Older adults may enjoy pantomiming famous people like former President Franklin Delano Roosevelt and his famous cigarette holder, the expressionless look of entertainer Jack Benny, or the "come hither" look of actress Hedy Lamar.

The next step would be to have clients suggest scenarios for mime. Some groups of clients may need prompting before developing a list of possible scenarios. Alcoholics may play a bartender refusing to sell a drunk another drink. Hospitalized clients may mime complaining to the dietitian about their food or to the orthotist about their appliance. Almost any concrete or intrapsychic problem can be mimed if clients think through exactly what message they wish to communicate. By paying attention to the details of communication, clients are often able to learn how they affect other people. Scenes can be replayed until the client or audience feels satisfied with the pantomime. In closing a mime session, clients may enact the various goodbye rituals we use—waving, hugging, or shaking hands (Straub, Straub, 1984; Alberts, 1971; Aubert, 1976; Blatner, 1973; Buchan, 1972; Corsini, Cardone, 1966; Gray, Percival, 1962; Weisberg, Wilder, 1985). Most clinics will not have the time to put on stage make-up for face painting for a mime session; however, if a group begins to elaborate its ideas and plan a performance, this may be an occasion to experiment with make-up or grease paint. Miming leads into other acting. Community centers offer opportunities and time to expand mime skills into more formal presentations (Wetherd, 1973).

MAGIC

Occupational therapists have been using magic as a medium of treatment for the last decade. Magic in many cases means the supernatural, casting a spell, or dark scary things we don't understand. For occupational therapy it is not supernatural or scary. It is a novelty for clients who have become bored with other types of treatment, such as repetitive exercise. *Project Magic* works to link therapists and magicians in order to facilitate their working together in teaching magic tricks to clients. They provide a trick book along with lists of local magicians who have an interest in working with clients. Tricks are used with one-handed clients, head trauma clients, or any clients who need to improve manual dexterity (Krinsky, 1998). In addition, there are a good number of books on magic that can be found in the juvenile section of the library (Milner, 1987b; Gibson, 1980; Lopshire, 1969; Severn, 1964, 1965, 1977; Waters, 1985). Tricks run the gamut from, for example, the magic penny in which the fledgling magician uses words to trick by saying, "I bet if I put down my penny you won't be able to jump over it," and then puts the penny down on top of the other person's head or shoulder (Gibson, 1980), to sophisticated card tricks. All tricks require practice to be performed smoothly (Milner, 1987b). Practice of difficult processes and movements are integral to client improvement of coordination, motor control, sequencing, and other cognitive components.

NONCOMPETITIVE GAMES

We have come to realize that cooperation compared to competition produces better performance outcomes. There has been a trend toward developing and using cooperative activities (Kohn, 1986; Rabow, 1988). In the 1970s, as the words *a happening* came to describe a group of people enjoying themselves together, occupational therapists began to use some of these *happening* activities with clients. Parachute games and Knots are two that are commonly used with many different kinds of clients (Orlich, 1978a; Martens, 1978; Fluegelman, 1976; French, Horvat, Alexander, 1983). Other cooperative game books soon followed for both children and adults (Fluegelman, 1981; Orlich, 1978b). The basic idea for all these activities is that people should be able to play together with each other, not against each other. When human energy is used against another, often someone gets hurt physically or psychologically. As the New Games Foundation motto asserts, "Play Hard, Play Fair, Nobody Hurt" (Fluegelman, 1976).

Some noncompetitive board games have also been used by occupational therapists for more than a decade. One such game is *The Ungame*. It is a values clarification game with decks of question cards, markers, and board positions. Originally, it had one model intended for all groups. Later, special decks of question cards were developed for children, all ages, and so forth (Zakich, 1983). It is the experience of the author that almost any diagnostic client group will enjoy *The Ungame*. *Slice of Life* is another board game for improving communication, self-image, leisure use, and time management (Michelson, 1985). For alcohol and drug abusers, *Sobriety* is a board game asking difficult questions about staying sober after discharge. For each of these games, literacy is almost a necessity. A therapist can adapt the rules so one person does all the reading to avoid putting an illiterate player on the spot. Each of these games is noncompetitive. Games have been developed to elicit family stories, reminiscence for the elderly, and to assist children in dealing with a variety of feelings from fears, sadness, and shyness, to cognitive performance components such as memory, logic, and problem solving.

An important point for the student of activities for occupational therapy is that there are new, exciting ideas for therapy being constantly developed. Because of the wide spectrum of available treatments, occupational therapists have a great deal of freedom in matching their client with appropriate activities.

REFERENCES

Alberts, D. (1971). *Pantomime: Elements and exercises.* Lawrence, KS: The University of Kansas Press.

Aubert, C. (1976). *The Art of pantomime.* New York: Arno Press.

Baygan, L. (1982). *Make-up for the theater, film and television.* New York: Drama Club Publishers.

Blatner, H. A. (1973). *Acting in: Practical applications of psychodramatic methods.* New York: Springer Publishing.

Buchan, L .G. (1972). *Roleplaying and the educable mentally retarded.* Belmont, CA: Fearon Publishers.

Buchman, L. G. (1975). *Stage makeup.* New York: Watson-Guptill Publications.

Corsini, R. J., & Cardone, S. (1966). *Roleplaying in psychotherapy.* Chicago: Aldine Publishing Company.

Fluegelman, A. (ed.). (1976). *The new games book.* Tiburon, CA: Headlands Press.

Fluegelman, A. (ed.). (1981). *More new games!* Tiburon, CA: Headlands Press.

French, R., Horvat, M., & Alexander, F. (1983). *Parachute movement activities-A complete parachute movement program for elementary school and beyond.* Byron, CA: Front Row Discovery.

Gibson, W. (1980). *Big book of magic for all ages.* Garden City, NY: Doubleday.

Gray, V., & Percival, R. (1962). *Music, movement and mime for children.* Toronto: Oxford.

Harris, S. M. (1985). *This is my trunk.* New York: Atheneum.

Harzberg, H., & Moss, A. (1924). *Slapstick and dumbell.* New York: Joseph Lawren.

Keysell, P. (1975). *Mime: Themes and motifs.* Boston: Plays, Inc. Publishers.

Kohn, A. (1986). *No contest.* New York: Houghton Mifflin.

Krinsky, R. (1998). Have you heard the news? *Advance for Occupational Therapists, 14*(2), 12,74.

Lopshire, R. (1969). *It's magic?* New York: MacMillan Publishing.

Martens, R. (1978). *Joy and sadness in children's sports.* Champaign, IL: Human Kinetics Publishers.

Michelson, B. (1985). *A slice of life.* DeKalb, IL.

Milner, M. (1987a). Actors avoid preaching to show lighter side of living with disability. *OT Week, 1*(2), 12-14.

Milner, M. (1987b). Occupational therapist and entertainer put magic into rehabilitation program. *OT Week, 1*(50), 12-13.

Orlich, T. (1978a). *The cooperative sports and games book: Challenge without competition.* New York: Pantheon Books.

Orlich, T. (1978b). *Winning through cooperation.* Washington DC: Acropolis Books, Ltd.

Pardoe, T. E. (1931). *Pantomimes for stage and study.* New York: Benjamin Bloom.

Phillips, M. E. (1996). The use of drama and puppetry in occupational therapy during the 1920s and 1930s. *Am J Occup Ther, 50*(3), 229-233.

Rabow, G. (1988). The cooperative edge. *Psychology Today, 22*(1), 54-58.

Severn, B. (1964). *Magic in your pockets.* New York: David McKay Company.

Severn, B. (1965). *Magic shows you can give.* New York: David McKay Company.

Severn, B. (1977). *Magic with coins and bills.* New York: David McKay Company.

Stolzenberg, M. (1981). *Clown for circus and stage.* New York: Sterling Publishing Co.

Straub, C., & Straub, M. (1984). *Mime: Basics for beginners.* Boston: Plays, Inc.

Waters, G. (1985). *Science tricks & magic.* London: Usborne Publishing Ltd.

Webster's Seventh New Collegiate Dictionary. (1969). Springfield, MA: G & C Merriam Company.

Weisberg, N., & Wilder, R. (1985). *Creative arts with older adults: A sourcebook.* New York: Human Sciences Press.

Wetherd, A. G. (1973). *Movement and drama in therapy.* Boston, MA: Boston Plays, Inc.

Zakich, R. (1983). *The ungame company.* Anaheim, CA.

APPENDICES

Vendors of Materials Described in this Text

AMACO
American Art Clay Company, Inc.
4717 West 16th Street
Indianapolis, Indiana 46222
1-800-374-1600
Fax 1-317-248-9300
catalog@amaco.com

Attainment Co. (instructional curricula for food preparation)
P.O. Box 930160
Verona, Wisconsin 53593
1-800-327-4269
Fax 1-800-942-3865
Infor@attainment-inc.com
http://www.attainment-inc.com

Craftime, Inc.
650 Ethel Street N.W.
P.O. Box 93706
Atlanta, Georgia 30377
1-800-849-8463
Fax 1-404-874-5148
craftime@mindspring.com
http://www.craftimeinc.com

Creative Crafts International
16 Plains Road
Essex, Connecticut 06426
1-800-854-5422
Fax 1-860-767-2904

Dick Blick Art Materials
P.O. Box 1267
695 Route 150
Galesburg, Illinois 61401-1267
1-800-447-8192
Fax 1-800-621-8293
info@dickblick.com
http://www.dickblick.com

HearthSong
P.O. Box 1773
Peoria, Il 61656-1773
1-800-325-2502
Fax 1-309-689-3857

MicroWarehouse (for computers and software)
1729 Oak Street
Lakewood, New Jersey 08701-5926
1-800-397-8508
Fax 1-732-942-2502
info1@warehouse.com

Mid-South Ceramic Supply Co.
1230 4th Avenue North
Nashville, Tennessee 37208
1-615-242-0300

MN Clay USA
8001 Grand Avenue South
Bloomington, Minnesota 55420
1-800-CLAY USA (252-9872)
Fax 1-612-884-1820
mnclayus@mm.com
http://www.mm.com/mnclayus/

Nasco Arts and Crafts
901 Janesville Avenue
P.O. Box 901
Fort Atkinson, Wisconsin 53538-0901
1-800-558-9595
Fax 1-920-563-8296

info@nascofa.com
http://www.nascofa.com

Queue, Inc. (Educational software and CD-ROMs)
338 Commerce Drive
Fairfield, Connecticut 06432
1-800-232-2224
Fax 1-203-336-2481
QUEUEINC@aol.com
http://home.cityqueue.com

Sammons Preston, Inc. (Adaptive equipment)
P.O. Box 5071
Bolingbrook, Illinois 60440-5071
1-800-323-5547
Fax 1-800-547-4333
sp@sammonspreston.com
http://www.sammonspreston.com

S & S Worldwide (Craft supplies and educational activities)
75 Mill Street
P.O. Box 513
Colchester, Connecticut 06415
1-800-243-9232
Fax 1-800-566-6678
rmflynn@snswwwide.com
http://www.snswwide.com

Sax Arts & Crafts
P.O. Box 510710
New Berlin, Wisconsin 53151
1-800-558-6696
Fax 1-800-328-4729
info@saxarts.com
http://www.saxarts.com

Smith & Nephew Roylan, Inc. (Adaptive equipment)
P. O. Box 1995 (for pre-paid orders or correspondence)
Germantown, WI 53022-8205
Or
P.O. Box 73276 (for invoice payments)
Chicago, Il 60673-7276
1-800-558-8633
Fax 1-800-545-7758

Tandy Leather Company
1400 Everman Parkway
Fort Worth, Texas 76140
1-817-551-9784
TCRAFTSL–CORP@TANDYCRAFTS.COM
http://www.tandyleather.com
Look in telephone book for local Tandy store number

Triarco Arts & Crafts
14650-28th Avenue North
Plymouth, Minnesota 55447
1-800-328-3360
Fax 1-612-559-2215

Unicorn Books and Crafts, Inc.
1338 Ross St.
Petaluma, California 94954
1-800-289-9276
unicorn@unicornbook.com

Vanguard Crafts, Inc.
1081 East 48 St.
P.O. Box 340170
Brooklyn, New York 11234
1-800-662-7238

ANNOTATED BIBLIOGRAPHY FOR CRAFTS

This appendix presents an annotated bibliography for the craft areas mentioned in this book. These references are different from the ones used in the text. Some are for the craftsperson who wishes for more advanced techniques, while others are a more thorough presentation of crafts described herein. Some are historical accounts of the craft's development. There is also a listing for specific cultural crafts, computer crafts, and one for other books on crafts for the clinic and for the handicapped. An asterisk (*) indicates a new addition to the bibliography in this edition of the book.

WOODWORKING

Woodcraft
By Bernard S. Mason
Cranbury, NJ: A. S. Barnes and Co., Inc., 1973.
Crafts for living in the woods, bark crafts, Indian and American pioneer woodcrafts, tools and games.

Arts and Crafts Objects Children Can Make for the Home
By Jean Lyon
West Nyack, NY: Parker Publishing Company, Inc., 1976.
A chapter on woodcraft techniques with lumber scraps for children.

The Complete Manual of Woodworking
By Albert Jackson, David Day and Simon Jennings
New York: Alfred A. Knopf, 1997.
A detailed guide to design techniques and tools for the beginner and expert. Has a glossary, index and excellent photos, drawings and explanations. Shows photos of various woods and describes their properties.

Shop-Tested Small Furniture You Can Make
By James E. Blume (ed.)
Des Moines, IA: Meredith Books, 1997.
Twenty-five projects for the skilled hobbiest. Accurate patterns.

The Complete Handbook of Power Tools
By George R. Drake
Reston, VA: Reston Publishing Company, Inc., 1975.
A complete presentation with photographs of most power tools used by occupational therapists, including precautions.

Amateur Craftman's Cyclopedia
By Popular Science Monthly
New York: Popular Science Publishing Company, Inc., 1937.
While most of this old how-to book is on woodcrafts, there are sections on electricity, radio, metal craft, photography, and weather measurement tools.

Woodworking
By Willis H. Wagner
South Holland, IL: The Goodheart-Willcox Co., Inc., 1975.
A basic text presenting power and hand tools. Shows how to do many small wood projects.

Easy Ways to Expert Woodworking
By Robert Scharff
New York: McGraw Hill Book Company, Inc., 1956.
Describes and has photos of most power shop tools and processes. Does not deal with hand tools. No project designs or plans.

Bench Woodwork
By John L. Feirer
Peoria, IL: C. A. Bennett Co., 1972.
Emphasis on handtools, though power tools are also presented. Plans for many projects are in the back.

How to Carve Wood: A Book of Projects and Techniques
By Richard Butz
Newton, CT: The Tauton Press, 1984.

Crosses the spectrum from simple to difficult. Has scale drawings, black and white photos, and an index.

*Chip Carving Patterns
By Wayne Barton
New York: Sterling Publishing Co., Inc., 1990.
Tells how to choose tools and materials. Has black and white photos, drawings, and an index. Includes simple patterns to those for the master carver.

Wood Carving and Whittling
by Popular Science Monthly
New York: Popular Science Publishing Company, Inc., 1936.
Thorough instructions for all kinds of carving.

LEATHERCRAFT

Leathercraft
By Fred W. Zimmerman
South Holland, IL: The Goodheart-Wilcox Co., Inc., 1969.
A basic book with traditional projects, designs, tools, and techniques.

Creative Leathercraft
By Grete Peterson
New York: Sterling Publishing Co., Inc., 1960.
A simple, small, well-illustrated book with many traditional projects but also leather embroidery and leather mosaic.

Leather Work Including Glove Making
By Albert H. Crampton
London: Frederick Warne & Co., Ltd.,1930.
An abbreviated description of tools and processes. It has a section on leather applique.

Modern Leather Design
By Don Willcox
New York: Watson-Guptill Publications, 1969.
Presents the process from rawhide to finished leather. Thorough presentation of tools, lacing, and tooling processes. Modern artistic designs for clothing, jewelry, furniture, and art.

Leathercraft
By Chris H. Groneman
Peoria, IL: Charles A Bennett Co., Inc., 1963.
A basic book with traditional small projects.

NEEDLEWORK

Arts and Crafts Objects Children Can Make for the Home
By Jean Lyon
West Nyack, NY: Parker Publishing Company, Inc., 1976.
A chapter on stitchery projects for both girls and boys.

Crafts for the Classroom
By Earl W. and Marlene M. Linderman
New York: MacMillan Publishing Co., Inc., 1977.
Easy-to-follow directions for many projects with children.

*The Good Housekeeping Illustrated Book of Needlecrafts
By Cecelia K. Toth (ed.)
New York: Hearst Books, 1994.
A compendium of knitting, crotchet, embroidery, needlepoint, quilting, and rug making. Excellent color photo illustrations.

*Reader's Digest Complete Book of Embroidery
By Melinda Cross
Pleasantville, NY: The Reader's Digest Association, Inc., 1996.
Contains an index, glossary, colored drawings, and photographs with patterns interspersed throughout the book. Excellent clarity of explanations.

Design in Fabric and Thread
By Aileen Murray
London: Watson-Guptill Publications, 1969.
Innovative designs for clothing, wallhangings, and other decorations. Many photographs in both color and black and white.

Classics for Needlepoint
By Susan Witt
Birmingham, AL: Oxmoor House, 1981.
Basic stitches, decorative stitches, bargello, and basketweave. Contains many designs and patterns.

120 Needlepoint Design Projects
By Barnes and David Blake
New York: Crown Publishers, Inc., 1974.
From types of canvas to dozens of designs.

Needlepoint Book
By Sylvia Sidney
New York: Van Nostrand Reinhold Company, 1968.
Contains an index of stitches and how to transfer designs.

Quilting as a Hobby
By Dorothy Brightbill
New York: Sterling Publishing Co., Inc., 1964.
A brief history. Describes trapunto, applique, and traditional American designs.

Quilting, Patchwork, Applique and Trapunto
By Thelma R. Newman
New York: Crown Publishers, Inc., 1974.
A book to stimulate artists. Photographs of historical and traditional works.

Knitting Without Tears
By Elizabeth Zimmerman
New York: Charles Scribrer's Sons, 1971.
From basic stitches to washing the sweater. Not enough pictures for beginners.

The Big Book of Knitting
By Isabelle Stevenson
New York: The Greystone Press, 1948.
Good diagrams and photos. Dozens of projects. Some complex decorative techniques.

Knitting Made Easy
By Barbara Aytes
Garden City, NY: Doubleday and Company, Inc., 1970.
Photographs are not easy to understand. For the advanced knitter, no matter what the title says.

COPPER AND METAL

Living Crafts
By George Bernard Hughes
Freeport, NY: Books for Libraries Press, 1954.
Contains four chapters on various metal crafts. Contains history as well as descriptions of 14 other crafts.

Arts and Crafts Objects Children Can Make for the Home
By Jean Lyon
West Nyack, NY: Parker Publishing Company, Inc., 1976.
Has a chapter on simple metal projects for children.

Metal Projects
By John R. Walker
South Holland, IL: The Goodheart-Wilcox Co., Inc., 1966.
Bending, welding, soldering, and riveting more than 50 projects.

Coppercraft and Silver Made at Home
By Karl Robert Kramer and Nora Kramer
Philadelphia: Chilton Company Book Division, 1957.
Thorough presentation of cutting, shaping, and riveting metal. Shows many possible projects.

*The Encyclopedia of Jewelry Making Techniques
By Jinks McGrath
Philadelphia: Running Press, 1995.
A comprehensive visual guide to traditional and contemporary techniques.
Excellent photos of 31 processes for making exquisite to playful jewelry. Shows shaping, forging, fusing, soldering, casting, and surface decorations for mostly metal jewelry and the tools required. Good index.

Fun With Colored Foil
By Manfred Burggraf
New York: Watson-Guptill Publications, 1969.
Good illustrations for cutting and shaping many decorative small projects.

MOSAICS

*Decorative Mosaics
By Elaine Goodwin
New York: Henry Holt & Co., 1992.
Well-illustrated history of the craft. Clear colored photographs of materials, tools, and techniques. Includes 14 projects, an index, and a short list of suppliers.

*Making Bits & Pieces: Mosaics
By Marlene Hurley Marshall
Pownal, VT: Storey Books, 1998.
Creative projects for home and garden. Tells how to use broken pottery, glass, buttons, and jewelry in constructing mosaics. Colored photographs of artists' work as well as how to do the projects. Good index.

*The Tile Decorating Book
By Marion Elliot
New York: Lorenz Books, 1997.
Includes a history of tiles with excellent photographs. Tells how to design and decorate ceramic as well as mosaic tiles. Many clear colored photographs of projects as well as techniques. Has an index and eight pages of patterns.

Modern Mosaic Techniques
By Janice Lovoos and Felice Paramore
New York: Watson-Guptill Publications, 1967.
For the artist. Wonderful photographs.

The Art of Making Mosaics
By Louisa Jenkins and Barbara Mills
Princeton, NJ: D. Van Nostrand Company, Inc., 1957.
Discusses materials. Has a chapter on children's mosaics and church art.

Mosaic Making
By Helen Hutton
New York: Reinhold Publishing Corporation, 1966.
Step-by-step presentation of various projects. How to
make, glaze and fire your own mosaic tiles.

Mosaics: Principles and Practice
By Joseph L. Young
New York: Reinhold Publishing Corporation, 1963.
Has some history. Many large mural-size projects.

Course in Making Mosaics
By Joseph L. Young
New York: Reinhold Publishing Corporation, 1956.
Contains a lot of information about of history. All black and white pictures.

CERAMICS

Crafts for the Classroom
By Earl W. and Marlene M. Lindermann
New York: MacMillan Publishing Co., Inc., 1977.
Simple clay and sculpture for the classroom.

*The Potter's Primer
By Morgen Hall
Iola, WI: Krause Publications, 1997.
Excellent photos of wedging, making slip, making molds, pouring molds,
combining clay of different colors, glazing, making tiles, and the processes of coil, slab, sgraffito, sculpture, and firing.

Glazes for the Potter
By William Ruscoe
New York: St. Martin's Press, 1974.
History of glazes. Complicated chemical formulas. Not for the beginner.

Making Pottery Without a Wheel
By F. Carlton Ball and Janice Lovoos
New York: Van Nostrand Reinhold Company, 1965.
Simple techniques and wonderful textures made from household items.

Fundamentals of Hobby Ceramics
By Bill Thompson
Livonia, MI: Scott Advertising and Publishing Co., 1975.
On pouring molds and numerous surface decoration techniques, some quite complex.

Introducing Handbuilt Pottery
By Tony Volly
New York: Watson-Guptill Publications, 1973.
Good photographs of simple and complex construction and decoration techniques. Artistic works.

The Self-Reliant Potter
By Andrew Holden
New York: Van Nostrand Reinhold Company, 1984.
For the rugged individualist who likes to make everything from scratch. A plan for how to get many materials for almost free in your own community.

Ceramics Techniques & Projects
By Elizabeth Hogan, supervising editor
Menlo Park, CA: Lane Magazine & Book Company, 1973.
Basic techniques for the hobby potter. Hand-building and wheel, no molds. Paper cover.

Pottery Designs
By David Close
London: B. T. Batsford, Ltd., 1984.
Photos and description of five basic techniques: slipware, pinch pots, slabs, modeling, and press molds.

Step-By-Step Ceramics
By Jolyen Hofsted
New York: Golden Press, 1967.
A well-illustrated introduction to basic principles and techniques. Photographs of stimulating designs. Paper cover.

WEAVING, LATCHOOK, MACRAMÉ, FIBERS

Arts and Crafts Objects Children Can Make for the Home
By Jean Lyon
West Nyack, NY: Parker Publishing Company Inc., 1976.
Has a chapter on simple weaving for children.

Crafts for the Classroom
By Earl W. and Marlene M. Lindermann
New York: MacMillan Publishing Co., Inc., 1977.
Thorough presentation of terms with simple directions for weaving and macrame.

Elements of Weaving
By Azalea Stuart Thorpe and Jack Lenor Larsen
Garden City, NY: Doubleday and Company, Inc., 1967.
Contains weaving history. Concentration on four-harness weaving.

Introducing Weaving
By Phyl Shillinglaw
New York: Watson-Guptill Publications, 1972.
Mostly simple looms. Presents dyes and various fibers.

Weaving Without a Loom
by Sarita R. Rainey
Worchester, MA: Davis Publications, Inc., 1972.
Includes God's eyes, paper, latchook, card weaving, and more. Pictures of artistic creations.

Weaving for Amateurs
by Helen Coates
London: The Studio Publications, 1946.
From small table loom, to four-harness loom, to dying, carding, and spinning.

*The Weaving, Spinning, and Dyeing Book, 2nd ed.
By Rachel Brown
New York: Alfred A. Knopf, 1995.
For the professional. Line drawings of various looms; inkle, backstrap, cardloom, ground loom, and floor loom. A few colored photographs of cloth. One hundred pages of suppliers, a glossary, and index.
Macramé and Other Projects for Knitting Without Needles
By Peggy Boehm
New York: Gramercy Publishing Company, 1963.
Ideas for many projects but diagrams are fuzzy.

Ojos de Dios: Eye of God
By Charles Albaum
New York: Grosset and Dunlap, 1972.
From the basics to complex tribal designs with illustrations and photographs.

Macramé
By Ann Stearns
New York: Arco Publishing Company, Inc., 1975.
Elaborate belts, jewelry, and clothes.

Fun With String
by Joseph Leeming
New York: Frederick A. Stokes Company, 1940.
Tricks and games, knots, macramé, braiding, handweaving, card weaving, and spool knitting. Good diagrams.

*Making Things: The Handbook of Creative Discovery
By Ann Sayre Wiseman
Boston: Little Brown and Co., 1997.
One hundred and twenty-five innovative projects for children, such as weaving, macramé, bread-dough sculpture, sandcasting, puppets, costumes, games, toys, and art. Illustrated with line drawings with color accents. Includes an index.

*Fun with Fabrics
By Juliet Bawden
New York: Random House, 1993.
Twenty-one different projects for children, from painting on fabrics to gluing, quilting, and stitchery.

PAPER CRAFTS

Arts and Crafts Objects Children Can Make for the Home
By Jean Lyon
West Nyack, NY: Parker Publishing Company Inc., 1976.
Has a chapter on simple paper projects for children.

*A Year of Crafts for Kids
By Kathy Ross
Brookfield, CT: Millbrook Press, 1996
Page after page of crafts organized by holidays, such as Earth Day, Hanukkah, Christmas, and Kwanzaa. Most crafts require about six common items like scissors, glue, tape, paint, a stapler, and paper or plastic containers. Each section has an introductory cultural explanation of the holiday. Bright color pictures show the process.

Crafts for the Classroom
By Earl W. and Marlene M. Linderman
New York: MacMillan Publishing Co., Inc., 1977.
Discusses developmental skills for art with children. Contains many paper projects for children.

*Papercraft: 50 Extraordinary Gifts & Projects, Step by Step
By Gillian Souter
New York: Crown Trade Paperbacks, 1997.
Colored photographs show papermaking, papier maché, paper weaving, paper folding, cut paper, sculpture, decoupage, and surface coloring techniques such as marbling, stenciling, and printing. Nice variety of crafts for a beginning clinic. Good index.

Modern Origami
By James Minoru Sakoda
New York: Simon and Schuster, 1969.
A nice progression from basic to complex origami.

*Classic Origami
By P.D. Tuyen
New York: Sterling Publishing Co., Inc., 1995.
Vietnamese author relates this art to his Vietnamese childhood. He discusses the origins of this craft and current trends. Thorough, clear sequential drawings of the process for the 26 animals which are listed in the index.

*Origami in Action: Paper Toys that Fly, Flap, Gobble, and Inflate
By Robert J. Lang
New York: St. Martins Griffin, 1997.
Sequential drawings of how to make 39 different figures. Each project is designated as easy, intermediate, or hard. A black and white photo shows the completed figure of each origami toy.

*Origami Animals
By Hector Rojas
New York: Sterling Publishing Company, Inc., 1993.
Wonderful photographs of real animals plus photographs of dioramas that include the origami animals. The book progresses from simpler to more complex projects. Some of the diagrams are small, which makes them more difficult to understand. This book is for the more accomplished paper folder.

Creative Origami
By Kunihiko Kasahara
London: Sir Issac Pitman and Son, Ltd., 1970.
Clear diagrams and photos of traditional forms as well as new artistic creations. One hundred different designs.

Art in Paper
By Carson I.A. Ritchie
South Brunswick: A. S. Barnes, 1976.
Includes silhouettes, decoupage, collage, paper sculpture, and oriental cut paper, as well as a short history on each topic.

The Paper Book: 187 Things to Make
By Don Munson and Allianora Rosse
New York: Charles Scribner's Sons, 1970.
Greeting cards, holiday decorations, dolls, costumes, buildings, and animals. Good diagrams and directions.

Paper Sculpture
by Tadeusz Lipski
London: The Studio, Ltd., 1947.
A small book. Simple to complex. Ten projects.

Paper Folding and Paper Sculpture
by Kenneth Ody
Buchanan, NY: Emerson Books, Inc., 1976.
A wide variety of uses of cutting, scoring, and folding. Good diagrams.

*The Art and Craft of Collage
By Simon Larbalestier
San Francisco: Chronicle Books, 1990.
Large color photographs of collages from dried flowers and greeting cards to plastic doll heads.

*Papier Mache' Style: 100 Step-by-Step Designs
By Alex MacCormick
Radnor, PA: Chilton Book Company, 1995.
Explains the history of this paper craft. Describes materials, processes for mold making, jewelry, papermaking, and finishes. Wonderful full-page photographs and an index. Has a list of English artists.

*The Art and Craft of Papier Maché
By Juliet Bowden
San Francisco: Chronicle Books, 1990.
Tells the history of paper mache' with photos of antique examples of the craft, folk art objects and modern papier maché art. Illustrations are

drawings of processes for making vessels, jewelry, whimsical sculptures, and decorator items. Has a list of English artists and a good index.

Creating With Corrugated Paper
By Rolf Hartung
New York: Reinhold Publishing, 1966.
Interesting designs, a maze, dolls, animals, vehicles, all from corrugated paper.

Paper People
By Michael Grater
New York: Taplinger Publishing Company, 1970.
Many toys, puppets, dolls, and novelties. Some period people.

COOKING

Creative Food Experiences for Children
By Mary T. Goodwin and Gerry Pollen
Washington D.C.: Center for Science in the Public Interest, 1974.
An easy-to-use format in this comprehensive cookbook for children, though the print is too small for children. Has nutrition information and ethnic foods.

Kitchen Classroom: Learning Through Cooking
By Shannon Wall-Mangum and Robin Franklin Matthew
Covington, LA: M and M Therapeutics, 1990.
This cooking curriculum by two occupational therapists has activities for teaching concepts related to cooking, food, and feelings about eating. Some worksheets can be copied for use.

*Better Homes and Gardens New Junior Cookbook
By Better Homes and Gardens Books
Des Moines, IA: Better Homes and Gardens, 1997.
Cartoon figures introduce sections on the basics of measuring, safety, menu planning, table-setting. Also includes a glossary and drawings of tools, pots, and pans. There are sections on the various meals and special foods such as desserts. The recipes take from two to eight steps, thus allowing for different levels of complexity.

*COMPUTER

*Kids' Computer Creations
By Carol Sabbeth
Charlotte VT: Williamson Publishing, 1995.
Explains computer functions from bytes to printer types. Many projects for ages 4 to 10 are shown and disucssed. Excellent even for adults begin-

ning to use graphics programs. It encourages exploration of drawing/painting possibilities while decreasing fear of failure. Includes some traditional crafts made from computer paper such as paper mache' projects.

Digital Magic with Microsoft: Picture It
By D.K.DeVerniero & Peter Kelly
Redmon, WA: Microsoft Press, 1997.
How to use photographs and images on home computers. Illustrates how to make photo collages.

Painter 5: Studio Secrets
By Adele Droblas Greenberg & Seth Greenberg
Foster City, CA: IDG Books Worldwide, Inc., 1998.
A compact disc is included with this book. Explanations begin with, "What is a pixel?" and move on to techniques for the most sophisticated artist.

Microsoft Image Composer for Dummies
By Brian Johnson
Foster City, CA: IDG Books Worldwide, Inc., 1998.
This guide starts with the most basic images and advances to web page design.

DRAWING AND PAINTING

Anyone Can Paint Pictures
by Alfred Paddy Kerr
New York: Pitman Publishing Corporation, 1960.
Simplified instructions for oil and watercolor painting. Most illustrations and pictures in black and white.

The Artist's Handbook of Materials and Techniques
by Richard Mayer
New York: The Viking Press, 1948.
Comprehensive for technical problems. Oils, tempera, watercolor, pastel crayons, pigment compositions, chemistry and murals.

The Artist's Handbook of Materials and Techniques, Revised Edition
By Ralph Mayer
New York: The Viking Press, 1957.
A classic manual for the studio artist. Comprehensive.

Weekend Painter
By Lawrence V. Burton
New York: Whittlesey House, 1948.
From basic color mixing to how to take criticism.

Oil Painting for the Beginner, Third Edition
By Frederic Taukes
New York: Watson-Guptill Publications, 1965.
Large print. Color perspectives, portraits, and landscapes.

The Creative Way to Draw Heads and Portraits
By Authur Zaidenberg
New York: Cornerstone LIbrary, 1969.
A step-by-step progression from simple lines, anatomy, separate facial features, shading, and special problems.

The Joy of Painting
By Arthur Zaidenberg
Garden City, New York: Hanover House, 1955.
Mostly human figure drawing and painting.

Introduction to the Visual Arts
By S. Ralph Maurello (Ed.)
New York: Tudor Publishing Company, 1968.
A basic description of art materials and a thorough, step-by-step course in the elements of drawing, color theory, perspective, decorative design, and other fundamentals of art. Well-illustrated with both color and black and white photographs.

*The Encyclopedia of Decorative Paint Techniques
By Simon Cavelle
Philadelphia: Running Press, 1994.
Covers most surface coloring techniques used in architecture, furniture finishes, trompe l'oeil, and accessories. Excellent photos of the process. Thorough index.

*Drawing with Children: A Creative Method for Adult Beginners, too
By Mona Brookes
New York: G. P. Putnam's Sons, 1996.
Gives consideration to environmental influences on the artist, on acquiring materials, on communicating with the child, appropriate activities for the developmental level, warm-ups and how to do still-lifes. Has black and white photos except one section of 64 small colored photos of drawings and paintings. This would be a good curriculum for a classroom.

*Drawing for Older Children & Teens: A Creative Method for the Adult Beginner, too
By Mona Brooks
New York: Jeremy P. Tarcher/Putnam, 1991.
For individuals from 8 years old to the adult beginner. Would be a good

classroom curriculum. Has 31 color photographs of artwork. All other illustrations are in black and white. Presents both positive and negative space concepts, as well as scale and perspective.

Painting for Children
    By Lois Thomasson Horne
New York: Reinhoid Book Corporation, 1968.
Gives basic materials, equipment, and techniques commonly used by teachers of children. Examples of paintings by age categories from 5 to 12 years old.

Finger Tip Magic: Theory and Practice in the Art of Finger Painting
By Margaret O'Brien
Springfield, MA: Milton Bradley Company, 1948.
An 18-page brochure with demonstration pictures of different techniques and effects.

Creating With Crayon
By Lothar Kampmann
New York: Reinhold Beck Corporation, 1967.
Techniques for using wax crayons. Wonderful color illustrations and examples of children's work. Good index.

*Paintcrafts
By Gillian Souter
New York: Crown Trade Paperbacks, 1997.
Fifty different gifts and projects with step-by-step instructions for marbleizing paper, making jewelry and gameboards, stenciling, fabric projects, stamping, painting on glass, ceramics, paper, and wood. Has an index and pages of patterns.

PRINTING

Elementary Screen Printing
By Albert Kosloff
Chicago, IL: Naz-dar Company, 1972.
A small book with a few illustrations. Describes the photographic process.

Screen Printing Process
By Albert Kosloff
Cincinnati, OH: The Signs of The Times Publishing Company, 1964.
A well-illustrated book with both commercial and studio printing described.

The Complete Book of Silk Screen Printing Production
By J. J. Biegeleisen
New York: Dover Publications, Inc., 1963.
Thorough with history, techniques, and products for the artist and commercial production.

The Art of the Print
By Fritz Eichenberg
New York: Harry N. Abrams, Inc., Publishers, 1976.
Reproduction of many masterpieces, history of all techniques, lengthy description of techniques.

Twentieth Century Graphics
By Jean Adhemar
New York: Praeger Publishers, 1971.
Mostly history. Little on how to do techniques.

The Art of Etching
By E. S. Lumsden
New York: Dover Publications, Inc., 1962.
A history and how-to book of drypoint etching, soft-ground etching, and aquatint. Thorough step-by-step presentation with illustrations.

*Nature Printing with Herbs, Fruits & Flowers
By Laura Donnelly Bethmann
Pownal, VT: Storey Publishing, 1996.
Includes many easy, yet innovative printing projects including how to print a spider web. Lovely color photos of materials and completed projects. Drawings show the process used.

*FOUND MATERIALS

*Cub Scout Leader How-to Book
By Boy Scouts of America
Irving, TX: Boy Scouts of America, 1994.
Has a 64-page chapter on crafts for boys 8 to 10 years of age. Excellent black and white drawings and patterns. Lists good sources for found materials. Also includes chapters on games, performance art, and outdoor nature activities. A thorough resource for boys' groups.

*Ecoart! Earth-Friendly Art & Craft Experiences for 3- to 9-year-olds
By Laurie Carlson
Charlotte, VT: Williamson Publishing, 1993.
Presents many tried and true simple crafts with new ideas in a new format. Ecological lessons are presented alongside the crafts. The black and

white line drawing are easily understood. Many products of nature ,such as seeds and pinecones, are used, as well as recycled plastic and paper discards. Good index.

Crafts in Minutes
By Susan Hernandez Ray and Adrienne E, Short (Eds.)
Birmingham, AL: Oxmoor House, 1997.
Has six categories of crafts: gifts, fashion, home décor, bazaar-type crafts, holidays and quick but clever ideas. The back has patterns for iron-ons and stencil making. Some good ideas for low and high functioning patients.

Trash to Treasure: The Recycler's Guide to Creative Crafts
By Anne Childs (Ed.)
Little Rock, AR: Leisure Arts, Inc., 1996.
How to give a second life to boxes, buckets, felt-pens, styrofoam packing, empty food containers, furniture, paper bags, pinecones, and vines. Seven pages of patterns for drawing or painting.

Beautiful Boxes
By Cheryl Owen
New York: Clarkson N. Potter, Inc./Publishers, 1996.
Shows 47 different boxes with a wide variety of techniques to decorate discarded boxes or boxes you buy, to make as gifts or storage. Good color photographs show techniques as well as finished products. Includes a glossary and index.

Naturecrafts
By Gillian Souter
New York: Crown Trade Paperbacks, 1996.
Fifty gifts and projects, step-by-step with an index, made from clay, reed/cane, twine, raffia, wax, flour and salt, fruit, flowers, shells, feathers, stones, sand, seedpods, and leaves.

The Complete Book of Gourd Craft
By Ginger Smith and Jim Widess
Ashville, NC: Lark Books, 1996.
Color photographs of completed projects and different types of gourds. Blank and white photographs show the processes involved. There are innovative ideas for 22 projects and 55 different decorative techniques.

ETHNIC OR CULTURE

Southwestern Arts and Crafts
By Nancy Krenz and Patricia Byrnes
Santa Fe, NM: The Sunstone Press, 1979.
Contains Mexican and Indian crafts, recipes, music, and dance for kindergarten through 6th grade.

The Kids' Multicultural Art Book
By Alexandra M. Terzian
Charlotte, VT: Williamson Publishing, 1993.
Twelve Native American tribal crafts, 15 Hispanic projects, 11 African crafts, and 12 Asian projects. Ingredients/supplies listed for each. Directions are given in numbered steps. Illustrations are line drawings. Has an index.

The Craftsman in America
By The National Geographic Society
Washington, D.C.: Special Publications Division, 1975.
Historic as well as modern crafts developed in America. Not a how-to book.

African Crafts and Craftsmen
By René Gardi
New York: Van Nostrand Reinhold Company, 1969.
Large print and wonderful photographs of a variety of crafts, from raw materials to finished products from across the African continent.

West African Weaving
By Venice Lamb
London: Gerald Duckworth and Co., Ltd., 1975.
Tribal maps show origins of various weaves. Many photos of weavers at work.

Classic Origami
By P. D. Tuyen
New York: Sterling Publishing Co., Inc., 1995.
Vietnamese author relates this art to his Vietnamese childhood. He discusses the origins of this craft and current trends. Thorough, clear sequential drawings of the process for the 26 animals that are listed in the index.

OTHER CRAFT BOOKS FOR THE DISABLED AND SPECIAL GROUPS

Arts and Crafts for Physically and Mentally Disabled
By Elaine and Loren Gould
Springfield, IL: Charles C. Thomas Publishers, 1978.
An extensive presentation of the implementation of craft programs for the disabled institutionalized client. It describes planning, coordinating, motivating, and utilizing patients, available space, time allocation, equipment, staff, personnel, and volunteers with detailed craft project descriptions.

Pastimes for the Patient, Revised Edition
By Marguerite Ickis
New York: A. S. Barnes and Co., Inc., 1966.
This text contains chapters on nature crafts such as plants, terrariums, bird crafts, chip carving, leather, drawing and painting, weaving and fibers, and music, as well as others.

Crafts for the Very Disabled and Handicapped
By Jane G. Kay
Springfield, IL: Charles C. Thomas, Publishers, 1977.
Many inexpensive and simple crafts. Decorations for both Jewish and Christian holidays.

Kits for Kids
By Nancy Towner Butterworth and Laura Peabody Broad
New York: St. Martin's Press, 1980.
Easy-to-read book of simple cratfs, projects, and gifts to make by children ages 3 years and up. Excellent index of crafts by type, skill level needed, and various group settings.

Accident Prevention Manual: For the Training Programs
Edited by Merle E. Strong
Madison, WI: American Technical Society, 1975.
Occupational Safety and Health Association laws, safety inspections, and reporting accidents.

How to Build Special Furniture and Equipment for Handicapped Children
By Ruth B. Hoffmann
Springfield, IL: Charles C. Thomas, Publisher, 1970.
Mostly about wood products such as standing boards, tables, chair equipment, creepers, etc.

Easy-to-Make-Aids for Your Handicapped Child
By Don Caston
Englewood Cliffs, NJ: Prentice-Hall Inc., 1981.
From measuring the child to buying supplies and construction of 40 projects.

Safety Manual: Ceramics
By AMACO
Indianapolis, IN: American Art Clay Co., Inc., 1988.
Covers all aspects of hazards in ceramics from clay, to glazes, to firing, to kiln wash. AMACO brand specific.

COMPLETED ACTIVITY/ OCCUPATIONAL ANALYSIS

The following is a sample completed activity/occupational analysis. The therapist can refer to it to determine what might be an appropriate response. On this activity analysis form, all performance components will be completed, although in actual practice a therapist might choose to do only one or two.

ACTIVITY/OCCUPATIONAL ANALYSIS

I. **Name of activity/occupation** *Tooling of a leather belt*

II. **Performance contexts** (for a hypothetical client)

  A. **Client's age/gender** *23/Male*

  B. **Diagnosis/disability status** *Drug addiction to alcohol with multiple uses of many other illegal drugs; peripheral neuropathy with weakness in all extremities.*

  C. **Residential environment** *Rural county alcohol and drug residential treatment center*

  D. **Family/friends situation** *Unmarried; estranged from parents, brothers and sisters due to alcohol problem.*

  E. **Ethnic/cultural identification** *Hispanic*

  F. **Economic/employment status** *Unskilled day laborer. No financial resources.*

  G. **Educational level** *10th grade*

  H. **Treatment setting** *Size of room: 30 x 15 feet with a 6 x 6-foot storage room for supplies. Working space per person: 30 square feet of floor space; 9 square feet of table surface. Furniture arrangement (use dia-*

gram if necessary): the clinic has 8 x 3-foot work table in a U-shaped arrangement. Lighting: normal indoor fluorescent lighting. Equipment and appliances: N/A. Ventilation and temperature: the occupational therapy clinic has a special vent and filter system to comply with institutional safety standards.

III. Treatment goal for which activity/occupation is intended *To enhance self-concept through completion of an attractive object valued in the Hispanic culture.*

IV. Materials and tools needed *Amount and cost of each: prices here are figured according to the 1998 institutional discount given to occupational therapy clinics.*

- *One 36 x 1 1/4-inch 8-oz. leather belt strip—$5.00*
- *One 4 x 3 1/2-inch rectangle of 5-oz. weight tooling leather—$1.00*
- *50 ft. of leather lace—$4.00*
- *Rectangular buckle blank for western-style buckle—$2.80*
- *Rotary punch—$40.00*
- *1in. oblong slotting punch—$10.00*
- *3-prong thonging chisel—$3.00*
- *Rawhide mallet—$14.00*
- *Swivel knife—$10.00*
- *Masonite tooling board—$4.00*
- *Skiver—$3.00*
- *Two pairs of rivets—10 cents*
- *Snap setter—$7.00*
- *Lacing needles—20 cents*
- *Belt design template—$3.00*
- *Tracing modeler—$4.00*
- *Edge creaser—$5.00*
- *Leather scissors—$24.00*
- *Utility knife—$4.00*

Stamping Tools:
- *Background tool—$3.80*
- *Beveler—$3.50*
- *Pear shader—$3.50*
- *Seeder—$3.30*
- *Mink oil finish—$4.00*
- *Sponge applicator—75 cents*

V. Pre-session preparation *Purchase materials. Cut belt strip from cowhide back.*

   A. By whom *Certified occupational therapy assistant (COTA).*
   B. Steps in preparation *Two.*
   C. Time required *Purchasing by telephone, 3 minutes, with 3-day wait for delivery. One-quarter hour to cut leather into belt strips.*

VI. Placement of tools and materials (i.e., in cupboard, on table) *In cupboard. Client must get his own materials and tools as directed by the therapist.*

VII. Steps in craft activity *(number in order and describe each step including time required)*

1. *Measure waist and mark leather length. (2 minutes)*
2. *Cut leather to correct length and shape end. Punch holes. Skive at fold. (15 minutes)*
3. *Cut two leather rectangles to fit buckle and cut slot for belt keeper and hole for prong. (10 minutes)*
4. *Wet leather with damp sponge and wait until it returns to natural color. (5 minutes)*
5. *Place template on leather.*
6. *Use tracing modeler to imprint leather. (15 minutes)*
7. *Mark belt edge with edge creaser. (5 minutes)*

End of session one and clean-up

8. *Allow leather to dry overnight.*
9. *Cut outline of design with swivel knife. (10 minutes)*
10. *Dampen leather with sponge. (1 minutes)*
11. *Bevel lines of design. (10 minutes)*
12. *Use background tool. (10 minutes)*
13. *Use pear shader and modeling spoon to contour leather. (15 minutes)*
14. *Use seeder to emphasize design.(5 minutes)*

End of session two and clean-up

15. *Cut slots for lacing buckle. (5 minutes)*
16. *Apply mink oil to grain side of belt strip and both sides of buckle. (15 minutes)*
17. *Allow to dry.*

End of session four and clean-up

18. *Lace buckle together using double cordovan lacing. (1 hour)*
19. *Rivet buckle to belt. (10 minutes)*

End of session five and clean-up

VIII. Method of instruction (i.e., demonstration, verbal directions, audio or visual aid) *Verbal directions as well as demonstration on scraps when necessary.*

IX. Opportunities for grading activity/occupation

A. Simpler to more complex *(1) Client can develop own design and trace it on; (2) can use greater variety of stamping tools.*

B. Complex to simpler *(1) Use picture stamps or alphabet letters; (2) a simple belt buckle rather than a leather-laced buckle.*

X. Precautions (i.e., balance/gait or suicidal risk) *Client could still have delirium tremens. Using sharp tools could be dangerous. Extremity weakness may need close observation during task by the therapist.*

XI. Performance Areas *Into which does this craft activity/occupation fall and why?*

    A. Health maintenance *Activity/occupation is at the center of health maintenance according to core occupational theory.*

    B. Home management *N/A*

    C. Care of others *Giving of a gift to his father could possibly be construed as "care for others" because it shows his caring.*

    D. Educational *N/A*

    E. Vocational/retirement (opportunities for practicing work-related skills)

        1. Taking instruction *Must take instruction from therapist.*

        2. Accepting authority *Must accept authority of therapist.*

        3. Being able to adapt *If design is not exactly what he wants he will need to adapt it.*

        4. Setting goals *Steps can be planned out with client at first session.*

        5. Planning and performing independently/cooperatively *He can plan independently if therapist discovers he is capable of it.*

        6. Practicing stress-management skills *If his time planning is off, he may need to manage stress related to time allowed in occupational therapy clinic before cleaning up.*

        7. Demonstrating good body mechanics *Awareness of or instruction in body mechanics may be required in bending over the table to wet the leather, imprint the leather, use the edge creaser, cut and tool the design and apply the finish.*

        8. Timing/waiting *Needs to wait two times for leather to dry.*

        9. Counting *Needs to measure length; count holes to punch.*

        10. Making decisions *Can decide on design, color, buckle design.*

        11. Self-evaluation *Can evaluate his performance outcome against initial plans and the actual belt against the clinic sample belt.*

F. Play/leisure exploration *Client identifies that leatherwork is a leisure activity he will enjoy in the future.*

G. Play leisure/performance *Client must realize that leatherwork cannot completely take the place of alcohol, that he must find other activities/occupations as well to have a well rounded life.*

XII. Performance components

    A. Sensorimotor

        1. Sensory awareness/processing

            a. Does the skin receive temperature and pressure stimulation during this craft?

            Yes, the client feels the cool, wet leather. Pressure into muscle and joint occurs while pressing the template unto the wet leather, edge creasing, during cutting with the swivel knife, beveling the design and hammering the stamping tools.

b. Is it essential to feel the relationship of body parts to each other for performance of this activity? (i.e., holding with one hand while pushing with palm of the other)

Yes, when measuring the waist, client must know where to measure. In bilateral movements, the client must be aware of where and when both extremities are to work together.

c. Does activity require that the client be able to distinguish the position and movement of the head during this activity? (i.e., bending over)

Only slightly in bending over the leather while tooling and hammering. The client is sitting most of the time.

d. Does the craft stimulate the visual system? How?

Yes, the client will see many designs before choosing.

e. Is the auditory system stimulated by this craft? How?

Yes, by the sounds made by the mallet and stamping tools.

f. Does the gustatory system receive stimulation? How?

N/A

g. Does the craft stimulate the olfactory system? How?

Yes, by the leather and the mink oil.

2. Perceptual Processing

a. Is stereognosis, knowing by feel, necessary during the process? When?

The activity can be done without it.

b. Is it necessary to be able to distinguish joint movement? Which joints?

Yes, client must be able to note finger and thumb flexion around tools, wrist and elbow and shoulder movements in hammering, finishing and lacing.

c. Does this craft cause any negative sensations? (i.e., pain, bad smells)

Hammering may cause too much auditory stimulation for some leather-workers. Some of the finishes have odors that may annoy.

d. Is awareness of body scheme or position of the body in space essential in this activity/occupation? When?

Yes, when measuring the waist size for the length of the belt.

e. Does the client need to discriminate the right from the left side in this craft? When?

Yes, in order to properly lace and attach the buckle with the design right side up and the belt lapping from left to the right side.

f. Is it necessary to discriminate whether forms, shapes and spaces are the same? When?

Yes, in choosing the right size of stamping tools and in choosing the correct size of slots for the size of needle to be used.

g. Will it be necessary to identify an incomplete object or picture in order to know how to complete this craft? (i.e., understand sequential diagrams in craft instructions)

Yes, if the client stops tooling between sessions one, two, or three. He needs to know what is incomplete in the design as well as which steps come next so he can proceed from there to finish.

h. Will it be necessary for the client to distinguish a figure or object from its background?

Yes, lacing requires the capability to see the lacing and distinguish it from the table on which the project lies. Choosing rivets requires selecting one from the background of the container. Tooling also requires focusing on the design foreground apart from the background.

i. Will the client be required to use depth perception to do this task? Explain.

Yes, depth perception is necessary to aim and judge the force needed in hammering, and in pressing in the design.

j. Is it necessary to distinguish the position of objects in relation to each other and/or to move from one object to another? Explain.

Yes, the position of the tooling implements and their movement are crucial to making the proper design. The position of the sponge in the water dish moving on to the leather is necessary. The lacing needle in relation to the holes for lacing is important.

B. Neuromusculoskeletal

1. Could the craft activity stimulate a reflexive movement? (i.e., loud noise causing client to jump)

Yes, hammering could cause the client to jump reflexively however it would be unusual for client to jump at their own hammering.

2. Which joint movements are involved? (i.e., flexion, extension, abduction, adduction)

a. Measuring: Finger flexion, thumb opposition, wrist flexion and extension; elbow flexion and extension; shoulder internal and external rotation, flexion, extension and scapular retraction.

b. Cutting leather: Cylindrical grasp, elbow flexion and extension, should extension. Punching holes-cylindrical grasp.

c. Cutting and slotting leather: Cylindrical grasp, wrist radial extension, elbow flexion and extension.

d. Wetting leather: Tip prehension, cylindrical grasp, elbow flexion and extension, should horizontal abduction.

e. Placing templates: Finger extensors and flexors.

f. & g. Imprinting leather and edge creasing: Finger flexion and extension, thumb opposition, wrist flexion and extension; elbow flexion and extension.

h. Using swivel knife: Modified 3-jaw chuck grasp, wrist radial and ulnar deviation.

i. Dampening leather: Thumb adduction, finger flexion and exten-

sion, wrist and elbow flexion and extension, shoulder horizontal abduction and adduction.

j. *Beveling: Finger and thumb-tip prehension, cylindrical grasp, wrist flexion and extension, forearm supination and pronation, elbow flexion and extension.*

k. *Background-Finger and thumb-tip prehension, cylindrical grasp, wrist flexion and extension, forearm supination and pronation, elbow flexion and extension.*

l. *Pear shader and modeling spoon: Finger and thumb-tip prehension, cylindrical grasp, wrist flexion and extension, forearm supination and pronation, elbow flexion and extension.*

m. *Seeder: Finger and thumb-tip prehension, cylindrical grasp, wrist flexion and extension, forearm supination and pronation, elbow flexion and extension.*

n. *Slot on buckle: Finger and thumb-tip prehension, cylindrical grasp, wrist flexion and extension, forearm supination and pronation, elbow flexion and extension.*

o. *Applying mink oil: Same as (i).*

p. *Lace buckle: Tip prehension and three-jaw chuck, wrist flexion and extension, forearm supination and pronation; elbow flexion and extension.*

q. *Riveting: Tip prehension, cylindrical grasp, wrist flexion and extension, forearm pronation and supination, elbow flexion and extension.*

3. Are movements passive or active?

Mostly active; a few passive motions due to gravity.

4. How much range of motion is necessary? (i.e., full, limited, moderate)

Full for hand, wrist and elbow; moderate for shoulder.

5. Is muscle tone limiting completion of task? (i.e., spasticity, flaccidity)

May be some muscle weakness and incoordination.

6. How will the client be positioned? (i.e., seated, standing, lying down)

Seated.

7. How much endurance and strength are required in each position?

One-hour sitting tolerance required; 15 to 25 pounds grip strength for the tools.

8. Does the client need to maintain upright posture?

Yes, as most motions cannot be made from stooped or reclining position.

C. Motor

1. Which of the muscle groups are involved?

Flexors, extensors of fingers 1-5, wrist, elbow and shoulder; thumb opposition; supinators/pronators of forearm; external and internal rotators of shoulder.

2. Is it necessary to move eyes or limbs across the midsagital line of the body?

Yes, when measuring for the length of the belt, hands and eyes cross the midline. When wetting the leather, using the edge creaser, hammering, and applying the finish.

3. Must both sides of the body work together?

Yes, when pressing the template with one hand while holding it in place with the other, while hammering, while lacing, while finishing the leather, both hands and arms are used together.

4. Does the craft require planning ahead before moving?

Yes, planning is required in order to move through each step as applying the template and the tooling are intricate and must be done in sequence to get the proper effect.

5. Is fine motor control or dexterity required?

Yes, dexterity is required for template application, carving the leather with the swivel knife, tooling, and lacing.

6. Must visual information be coordinated with body movement?

Yes, client must be able to see the lines through the template in order to press in the correct place to get an imprint. The client's eyesight must be adequate to see where to place the ends of the stamping tools in the proper line or section. Vision is important in hitting the head of the stamping tools. Eye-hand coordination are necessary for lacing.

D. Cognition

1. Orientation (Is each of the below necessary? Why?)

a. Time: *Yes, to arrive at occupational therapy on time.*

b. Place: *Yes, to know how to find occupational therapy clinic.*

c. Person: *Yes, to know why he can benefit from this activity.*

2. Recognition (able to identify things previously presented)

Client must recognize where he stopped the previous session. He must recognize the stamping tools used to get the correct design. He must recognize which steps comes next.

3. Memory

a. Short-term memory requirements (10 seconds to 10 minutes)

Necessary to follow oral instructions.

b. Recent memory requirements (hours, days, months)

Necessary to remember where he stopped on previous day.

c. Long-term memory requirements (years to remote past)

Not necessary.

4. Attention span (longest period of time required for concentrating on one step)

1 hour

5. Initiating and terminating an activity appropriately

Client must know when a process is finished and when to start the next step.

6. Sequencing actions in the correct order

This is absolutely necessary to get a good design and a functional belt.

7. Mentally manipulating objects spatially

The client must understand that the design on the belt will appear as a mirror image of the design on the template. It is necessary to be able to imagine how to put the needle through the lace and through the hole as well as how to rivet the buckle to the belt so it will open the right way.

8. Problem solving

a. Recognizing existence of problem

Client must recognize when leather is too wet, when cutting and tooling are too deep or shallow, when lacing is irregular, when leather finish is too thick.

b. Think of a solution

Client can think of how to dry leather more quickly, how to better gauge depth of cut or stroke, how to wipe off excess finish.

c. Implement and evaluate the solution

Client may develop techniques to resolve the problems described in (a).

9. Can the client use elsewhere what is learned in doing this craft?

This client can learn the benefits of waiting till the leather is the right dryness for continued work or applying finish.

E. Psychosocial

1. Does the craft provide opportunity to discover what is valuable to client?

Yes, he is reconnected with the status of good, tooled leather in the Hispanic culture and for himself.

2. Is the client interested enough to pay attention for the length of time required to do the craft?

Yes, the client is very motivated to complete this project

3. Could the craft contribute to self-esteem?

Yes, his self-esteem is positively affected and client may be praised by other patients and therapist on work. This is the treatment goal toward which this particular craft is directed.

4. Does the craft reinforce the client's roles and/or gender identity?

It reinforces his gender identity as a Hispanic male because nicely tooled belts are highly valued for men in the Mexican-American culture.

5. Is the practice of social skills necessary to complete the craft? (i.e., prefacing requests with please)

The client must ask for appropriate assistance and guidance from the therapist, say please and thank you. Other patients may be using some of the same tools and client may need to use social skills in sharing them.

6. What communication will be required?

a. By the client: *Requests for assistance, receptivity to oral instructions from therapist.*

    b. By the therapist: *Capability to give clear instructions and to supervise activity/occupation without interjecting herself into the patients' work.*

    c. By another client: *May need to request tools used by the client, or to wait to ask for help as soon as therapist is free.*

    d. With the group: *The therapist may need to clarify for the group which tools and space will need to be shared.*

7. Does craft offer opportunities for affective expression?

a. Hostility/aggression (i.e., motions such as hammering, tearing, piercing)

Yes, hammering, pressing with spoon, cutting.

b. Sadness (i.e., slow movements)

Wiping can be slow and rhythmical.

c. Happiness (i.e., pride, hope, laughter)

Can express ethnic pride through choice of design, through completion of an esthetically pleasing item.

d. Loving (i.e., stroking, holding)

Wiping on water and oil.

8. Does craft provide opportunities for testing reality of client's own perceptions/beliefs (i.e., is my behavior/perception/belief normal?)

Yes, if client asks for therapist's evaluation of his performance and craftsmanship, it could validate or invalidate self-perception. Client will receive direct feedback from the efficacy of his work to test his own perceptions.

9. What impulse control is necessary?

The client must cooperate with time schedule of therapist and use tools safely. The client must exercise impulse control to prevent skipping steps, to prevent working on wet leather when it should be dry and visa versa, and from tooling too quickly in a slap-dash fashion.

10. Is there an opportunity to develop leadership skills while doing the craft?

This could lead to client being able to instruct other patients on a similar project.

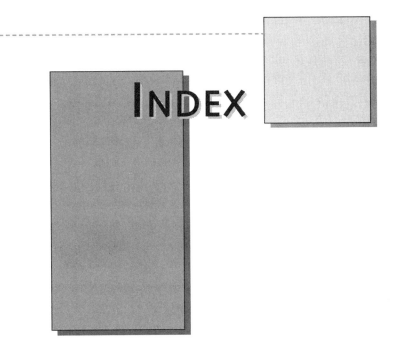

INDEX

For your information

This book and many others on numerous different topics are available from SLACK Incorporated. For further information or a copy of our latest catalog, contact us at:

Professional Book Division
SLACK Incorporated
6900 Grove Road
Thorofare, NJ 08086 USA
Telephone: 1-609-848-1000
1-800-257-8290
Fax: 1-609-853-5991
E-mail: orders@slackinc.com
WWW: http://www.slackinc.com

We accept most major credit cards and checks or money orders in US dollars drawn on a US bank. Most orders are shipped within 72 hours.

Contact us for information on recent releases, forthcoming titles, and bestsellers. If you have a comment about this title or see a need for a new book, direct your correspondence to the Editorial Director at the above address.

*If you are an instructor, we can be reached at the address listed above or on the Internet at **educomps@slackinc.com** for specific needs.*

Thank you for your interest and we hope you found this work beneficial.